BIOCHEMISTRY

(AS PER PCI, NEW DELHI FOR THE STUDENTS OF B. PHARM 2ND SEMESTER)

Mrs. Blessy Jacob
Associate Professor
T. John College of Pharmacy, Bengaluru,
Karnataka

Dr. Sarita Karole
Director
IQAC, at Oriental Institute of Pharmacy and Research,
Bhopal, M.P.

Prashant
Assistant Professor
F.S. University, Shikohabad, Firozabad, U.P.

Jyoti Sharma
Lecturer
Smt. Mahadevi College of Pharmacy,
Shikohabad, Firozabad, U.P.

SAMANT PUBLISHING

ISBN : 9788169244459
Edition : First, April 2026
Title : Biochemistry
Author : Mrs. Blessy Jacob, Dr. Sarita Karole, Prashant, Jyoti Sharma

Published by

SAMANT PUBLISHING

An Imprint of **Taneesha and Prachi NextGen Publication**

Plot No. 48, Khasra No. 646, Road No. 2,
Suman Nagar, Haridwar, Uttarakhand – 249402, India
Website : www.samantpublishing.com
E-mail : support@tpnextpub.com
Phone : +91 9760418103

Printed by :
Manipal Technologies Limited, Bengaluru - 560001, Karnataka

INDEX

Chapter-1

Biomolecules

Biomolecules are organic compounds produced by living organisms and are essential for the growth, development, maintenance, and regulation of physiological functions. They include a wide range of substances such as carbohydrates, proteins, lipids, nucleic acids, vitamins, and minerals, each performing specific and vital roles in the body. These molecules interact in a highly organized and regulated manner to support cellular structure, energy production, enzymatic reactions, genetic information storage, and signal transduction.

From a pharmaceutical perspective, an understanding of biomolecules is crucial because most drugs interact directly or indirectly with these molecules. Enzymes act as drug targets, proteins serve as receptors, carbohydrates and lipids participate in cell recognition and membrane integrity, and nucleic acids are involved in genetic regulation and therapeutic interventions. Knowledge of biomolecular structure and function helps in understanding drug absorption, distribution, metabolism, and excretion, as well as the biochemical basis of diseases.

Classification of Biomolecules

Biomolecules are classified based on their chemical nature, molecular complexity, and biological functions. This classification helps in understanding their structural characteristics, metabolic roles, and importance in living systems. In living organisms, biomolecules are broadly categorized into inorganic and organic biomolecules, each playing essential roles in maintaining life processes.

1.Inorganic Biomolecules

Inorganic biomolecules include substances that do not contain carbon-hydrogen bonds but are vital for normal physiological functions. Water is the most abundant inorganic biomolecule in living systems and serves as a universal solvent, reaction medium, and regulator of body temperature. It participates directly in biochemical reactions such as hydrolysis and condensation. Minerals and electrolytes, such as sodium, potassium, calcium, magnesium, chloride, phosphate, and iron, are also inorganic biomolecules. They are required for maintaining osmotic balance, nerve impulse transmission, muscle contraction, enzyme activation, bone formation, and oxygen transport. Although required in small quantities, their absence or imbalance can lead to serious metabolic and physiological disorders.

2.Organic Biomolecules

Organic biomolecules are carbon-containing compounds synthesized by living organisms. These molecules form the structural and functional framework of cells and tissues and are directly involved in metabolic activities. Organic biomolecules are further classified into carbohydrates, lipids, proteins, nucleic acids, and other biologically important compounds such as vitamins and enzymes.

a. Carbohydrates

Carbohydrates are polyhydroxy aldehydes or ketones or substances that yield such compounds on hydrolysis. They are primarily composed of carbon, hydrogen, and oxygen. Carbohydrates serve as the major source of energy for living organisms and are also involved in structural functions, cell recognition, and metabolic regulation. Examples include glucose, starch, glycogen, and cellulose.

b. Lipids

Lipids are a diverse group of hydrophobic or amphipathic organic compounds that are insoluble in water but soluble in organic solvents. They include fats, oils, waxes, phospholipids, glycolipids, and steroids. Lipids act as concentrated energy reserves, components of cell membranes, insulators, and precursors of hormones and bile acids.

c. Proteins

Proteins are complex organic molecules composed of amino acids linked by peptide bonds. They are the most abundant and functionally diverse biomolecules in living systems. Proteins perform structural, catalytic, transport, regulatory, protective, and contractile functions. Enzymes, antibodies, hormones, and receptors are all protein in nature, making proteins highly significant in pharmaceutical sciences.

d.Nucleic Acids

Nucleic acids are polymers of nucleotides and are responsible for the storage, transmission, and expression of genetic information. The two main types of nucleic acids are deoxyribonucleic acid (DNA) and ribonucleic acid (RNA). DNA carries hereditary information, while RNA plays a crucial role in protein synthesis and gene regulation.

d. Vitamins

Vitamins are organic compounds required in small quantities for normal growth and metabolic functions. They act mainly as coenzymes or precursors of coenzymes in various biochemical reactions. Vitamins are classified as fat-soluble and water-soluble, and their deficiency leads to specific deficiency disorders.

3.Based on Molecular Complexity

Biomolecules can also be classified into small biomolecules and macromolecules. Small biomolecules include monosaccharides, amino acids, fatty acids, nucleotides, and vitamins, which serve as building blocks. Macromolecules include polysaccharides, proteins, nucleic acids, and complex lipids formed by the polymerization of small biomolecules. This classification highlights the hierarchical organization of biomolecules in living systems.

Chemical Nature of Carbohydrates

Carbohydrates are organic compounds composed primarily of carbon, hydrogen, and oxygen, with hydrogen and oxygen generally present in the ratio of 2:1, similar to water. Chemically, carbohydrates are defined as polyhydroxy aldehydes or ketones, or substances that yield such compounds on hydrolysis. The basic chemical structure of carbohydrates consists of one or more hydroxyl (–OH) groups and a carbonyl group, which may be an aldehyde group (–CHO) as in aldoses or a ketone group (>C=O) as in ketoses. The simplest carbohydrates are monosaccharides, which cannot be hydrolyzed into simpler sugars and usually contain three to seven carbon atoms. These monosaccharides may exist in open-chain or cyclic ring forms in aqueous solutions due to internal hemiacetal or hemiketal formation. Monosaccharide units are linked together by glycosidic bonds to form disaccharides, oligosaccharides, and polysaccharides. Polysaccharides may be linear or branched polymers of monosaccharide units and serve either storage or structural functions. Carbohydrates may also occur as conjugated molecules such as glycoproteins, glycolipids, and proteoglycans, where carbohydrate moieties are covalently linked to proteins or lipids, contributing to their chemical and biological properties.

Biological Role of Carbohydrates

Source of Energy: Carbohydrates are the primary source of energy in the body. Glucose is the main energy-yielding carbohydrate and is essential for normal functioning of the brain and red blood cells.

Energy Storage: Excess carbohydrates are stored as glycogen in animals and starch in plants, serving as an energy reserve.

Structural Role: Carbohydrates provide structural support, such as cellulose in plant cell walls and glycosaminoglycans in connective tissues.

Cell Recognition and Immunity: Carbohydrates on cell surfaces play an important role in cell recognition, blood group determination, and immune responses.

Regulatory and Protective Functions: They are components of nucleic acids and mucopolysaccharides, contributing to genetic functions, lubrication, and protection of tissues.

Chemical Nature of Lipids

Lipids are a heterogeneous group of organic compounds that are generally insoluble in water but soluble in non-polar organic solvents such as ether, chloroform, and benzene. Chemically, lipids are composed mainly of carbon, hydrogen, and oxygen, and in some classes may also contain phosphorus, nitrogen, sulfur, or other elements. Unlike carbohydrates and proteins, lipids are not true polymers, but they are characterized by the presence of long hydrocarbon chains or ring structures that confer hydrophobic properties. The basic building blocks of many lipids are fatty acids, which are long-chain carboxylic acids that may be saturated or unsaturated. Fatty acids are commonly esterified with alcohols such as glycerol to form complex lipids.

Simple lipids include fats and oils, which are chemically triacylglycerols formed by the esterification of three fatty acid molecules with one glycerol molecule. Compound lipids contain additional groups besides fatty acids and glycerol, such as phospholipids, glycolipids, and lipoproteins. Phospholipids contain a phosphate group and are amphipathic in nature, possessing both hydrophilic and hydrophobic regions. Derived lipids are substances obtained from the hydrolysis of simple and compound lipids and include fatty acids, sterols such as cholesterol, fat-soluble vitamins, and hormones. Lipids may exist in different physical forms depending on the degree of saturation of fatty acids and play a key role in forming biological membranes due to their chemical structure.

Biological Role of Lipids

Source of Energy: Lipids serve as a concentrated source of energy, providing more energy per gram than carbohydrates or proteins. They act as long-term energy reserves in adipose tissue.

Structural Role: Lipids are essential components of biological membranes. Phospholipids and cholesterol form the structural framework of cell membranes and maintain membrane fluidity and integrity.

Protective and Insulating Function: Lipids provide thermal insulation and mechanical protection to vital organs. Adipose tissue cushions organs and helps maintain body temperature.

Role in Hormone and Vitamin Function: Certain lipids act as precursors for steroid hormones, bile acids, and prostaglandins. Lipids are also necessary for the absorption and transport of fat-soluble vitamins A, D, E, and K.

Regulatory and Metabolic Functions: Lipids play an important role in cell signaling and regulation of metabolic processes. They are involved in nerve conduction and brain function due to their high concentration in nervous tissue.

Chemical Nature of Nucleic Acids

Nucleic acids are high-molecular-weight biomolecules that function as the carriers of genetic information in all living organisms. Chemically, they are polymers composed of repeating units called nucleotides. Each nucleotide consists of three essential components: a nitrogenous base, a pentose sugar, and a phosphate group. The nitrogenous bases are of two types, purines and pyrimidines. Purines include adenine and guanine, while pyrimidines include cytosine, thymine, and uracil. The pentose sugar is ribose in ribonucleic acid (RNA) and deoxyribose in deoxyribonucleic acid (DNA). The phosphate group links the sugar molecules of adjacent nucleotides, forming a sugar-phosphate backbone.

Nucleotides are linked together by phosphodiester bonds between the 3′ hydroxyl group of one sugar and the 5′ phosphate group of the next nucleotide, resulting in a polynucleotide chain. DNA typically exists as a double-stranded helical structure, with two antiparallel strands held together by hydrogen bonds between complementary base pairs, adenine pairing with thymine and guanine pairing with cytosine. RNA is usually single-stranded and may fold into complex secondary and tertiary structures. Due to the presence of negatively charged phosphate groups, nucleic acids are acidic in nature and exhibit polyanionic properties at physiological pH.

Biological Role of Nucleic Acids

Storage of Genetic Information: The primary biological role of nucleic acids is the storage of genetic information. DNA contains the hereditary material that determines the structure, function, and characteristics of an organism and is transmitted from one generation to the next.

Protein Synthesis: Nucleic acids play a central role in protein synthesis. DNA directs the synthesis of messenger RNA through transcription, and RNA molecules such as mRNA, tRNA, and rRNA participate in the translation of genetic information into specific proteins essential for cellular structure and function.

Regulation of Cellular Activities: Nucleic acids regulate cellular metabolism and activities by controlling enzyme synthesis and protein production. Through gene expression and regulation, they influence cell growth, differentiation, and adaptation.

Role in Cell Division and Inheritance: During cell division, DNA replicates accurately to ensure that genetic information is equally distributed to daughter cells. This process is essential for growth, tissue repair, and reproduction.

Metabolic and Structural Functions: Certain nucleotides and their derivatives function as energy carriers and coenzymes, such as adenosine triphosphate, nicotinamide adenine dinucleotide, and flavin adenine dinucleotide. These compounds play vital roles in energy transfer and metabolic reactions.

Chemical Nature of Amino Acids

Amino acids are organic compounds that serve as the fundamental structural units of proteins. Chemically, amino acids contain both an amino group ($-NH_2$) and a carboxyl group ($-COOH$) attached to the same carbon atom known as the α-carbon. In addition to these two functional groups, the α-carbon is bonded to a hydrogen atom and a variable side chain or R-group, which differs for each amino acid and determines its chemical properties and biological behavior. Most naturally occurring amino acids in proteins are α-amino acids and exist in the L-configuration. At physiological pH, amino acids exist as zwitterions, carrying both a positive charge on the amino group and a negative charge on the carboxyl group, which contributes to their amphoteric nature and buffering capacity.

Based on the chemical nature of their side chains, amino acids may be classified as non-polar, polar uncharged, acidic, or basic. Some amino acids contain additional functional groups such as hydroxyl, sulfhydryl, amide, or aromatic rings, which influence their reactivity and interactions. Amino acids are linked together by peptide bonds formed between the carboxyl group of one amino acid and the amino group of another, resulting in the formation of peptides and proteins. The sequence and composition of amino acids in a protein determine its three-dimensional structure and biological function.

Biological Role of Amino Acids

Building Blocks of Proteins: The primary biological role of amino acids is to serve as the building blocks of proteins. Proteins perform a wide range of functions, including enzymatic catalysis, structural support, transport, regulation, and immune defense.

Role in Metabolism and Energy Production: Amino acids participate in metabolic pathways and can be used as a source of energy when carbohydrates and fats are insufficient. They also act as intermediates in various biosynthetic processes.

Precursor of Biologically Important Compounds: Several amino acids serve as precursors for important biomolecules such as neurotransmitters, hormones, nucleotides, heme, creatine, and nitric oxide, playing crucial roles in physiological regulation.

Regulation of Acid–Base Balance: Due to their amphoteric nature, amino acids help maintain acid–base balance in the body by acting as buffers in physiological systems.

Role in Growth and Tissue Repair: Amino acids are essential for growth, development, and repair of body tissues. Essential amino acids must be supplied through the diet as they cannot be synthesized by the human body.

Chemical Nature of Proteins

Proteins are large, complex macromolecules composed of one or more linear chains of amino acids, which are linked together by covalent peptide bonds. Chemically, a protein is a polypeptide in which the amino acids are connected through a condensation reaction between the carboxyl group (–COOH) of one amino acid and the amino group (–NH_2) of another, forming a peptide bond (–CO–NH–). The sequence of amino acids in the polypeptide chain, known as the primary structure, determines the protein's overall structure and function. Proteins are amphoteric in nature due to the presence of ionizable groups such as amino and carboxyl groups, allowing them to act as buffers at physiological pH.

Proteins exhibit multiple levels of structural organization. The secondary structure arises from hydrogen bonding between backbone atoms, forming α-helices or β-pleated sheets. The tertiary structure refers to the three-dimensional folding of a single polypeptide chain stabilized by hydrogen bonds, ionic interactions, hydrophobic interactions, and disulfide bridges. Quaternary structure is observed in proteins composed of more than one polypeptide chain, where multiple subunits assemble to form a functional protein complex. Proteins may also be simple, consisting only of amino acids, or conjugated, containing non-protein components such as carbohydrates (glycoproteins), lipids (lipoproteins), metals (metalloproteins), or heme groups (hemoproteins).

Biological Role of Proteins

Structural Function: Proteins provide structural support to cells and tissues. Examples include collagen in connective tissues, keratin in hair and nails, and elastin in ligaments.

Enzymatic and Catalytic Role: Many proteins function as enzymes, catalyzing biochemical reactions with high specificity and efficiency, which is essential for metabolism and cellular processes.

Transport and Storage: Proteins facilitate the transport of molecules across membranes and within the bloodstream. Hemoglobin transports oxygen, while ferritin stores iron in the body.

Regulatory Function: Proteins act as hormones and signaling molecules that regulate physiological processes. Examples include insulin, glucagon, and growth hormone.

Defense Mechanisms: Proteins are involved in immune defense. Antibodies (immunoglobulins) protect the body against pathogens, while complement proteins assist in immune responses.

Energy Source: Although carbohydrates and lipids are the primary energy sources, proteins can be metabolized for energy during prolonged fasting or starvation.

Role in Growth and Repair: Proteins are essential for tissue growth, repair, and maintenance, providing the necessary amino acids for new cell synthesis.

Chapter-2

Bioenergetics

Bioenergetics is a specialized branch of biochemistry that deals with the study of energy flow and transformation in biological systems. It focuses on how living organisms acquire, convert, and utilize energy to sustain life processes. All cellular activities, including growth, reproduction, movement, and maintenance of homeostasis, require energy. Bioenergetics provides a framework to understand these processes at the molecular and cellular levels by studying the thermodynamic principles governing biochemical reactions.

The primary source of energy in biological systems is derived from the breakdown of nutrients such as carbohydrates, lipids, and proteins. This energy is captured in the form of high-energy molecules like adenosine triphosphate (ATP), which acts as the universal energy currency of the cell. Bioenergetics also examines the efficiency of energy conversion, the coupling of exergonic (energy-releasing) and endergonic (energy-requiring) reactions, and the role of enzymes in facilitating these transformations.

Furthermore, bioenergetics integrates concepts from chemistry, physics, and biology to explain how energy gradients, such as proton gradients across membranes, drive essential processes like oxidative phosphorylation and ATP synthesis. Understanding bioenergetics is fundamental in areas like metabolism, pharmacology, physiology, and clinical sciences, as it provides insight into how energy imbalances can lead to diseases and how therapeutic interventions can restore cellular energy homeostasis.

Concept of Free Energy

Free energy is a central concept in bioenergetics that helps quantify the energy available to do work in biochemical reactions. In living systems, not all energy released during a reaction is usable; some is lost as heat. Free energy specifically refers to the portion of total energy in a system that can perform useful work at constant temperature and pressure. It is represented by the symbol **G**, known as Gibbs free energy.

Gibbs Free Energy (G): Gibbs free energy combines enthalpy (total heat content, H), entropy (degree of disorder, S), and temperature (T) into a single value that indicates whether a reaction can occur spontaneously. The change in Gibbs free energy during a reaction is expressed as:

$$\Delta G = \Delta H - T\Delta S$$

Where:

- **ΔG** = Change in Gibbs free energy
- **ΔH** = Change in enthalpy (heat content)
- **T** = Absolute temperature in Kelvin
- **ΔS** = Change in entropy

Interpretation of ΔG:

- **ΔG < 0 (Negative ΔG):** The reaction is **spontaneous** and can proceed without external energy input. Such reactions are called **exergonic reactions**.
- **ΔG > 0 (Positive ΔG):** The reaction is **non-spontaneous** and requires input of energy to proceed. These are **endergonic reactions**.
- **ΔG = 0:** The system is at **equilibrium**, and no net energy is available to do work.

Standard Free Energy Change (ΔG°): This is the change in Gibbs free energy under standard conditions, which include 1 M concentration of reactants and products, 1 atm pressure, and 25°C temperature. Standard free energy is often used to compare the energy changes of different biochemical reactions.

Coupling of Reactions: In biological systems, endergonic reactions, which require energy, are often coupled with exergonic reactions, such as the hydrolysis of ATP, to make the overall process spontaneous. This coupling is essential for processes like biosynthesis, active transport, and muscle contraction.

Biological Significance of Free Energy: Understanding free energy changes allows biochemists to predict the direction of metabolic reactions, evaluate reaction spontaneity, and design pathways that efficiently harness cellular energy. It also helps in understanding energy transduction mechanisms, including oxidative phosphorylation and photosynthesis, where chemical energy is converted into usable cellular energy.

Endergonic and Exergonic Reactions

In bioenergetics, biochemical reactions are classified based on the change in free energy (ΔG) during the reaction. Understanding whether a reaction absorbs or releases energy is crucial for comprehending cellular metabolism and energy flow.

a. Exergonic Reactions: Exergonic reactions are reactions that **release free energy** and occur spontaneously under standard physiological conditions. In these reactions, the free energy of the products is lower than that of the reactants, resulting in a **negative ΔG ($\Delta G < 0$)**. Because energy is released, exergonic reactions can drive other biochemical processes, especially those that require energy.

Characteristics of Exergonic Reactions

- ΔG is negative ($\Delta G < 0$).
- Energy is released during the reaction.
- Reaction occurs spontaneously.
- Often coupled to endergonic reactions in cells to drive energy-requiring processes.

Examples

- Hydrolysis of ATP to ADP and inorganic phosphate (ATP $\rightarrow$ ADP + Pi).
- Breakdown of glucose in glycolysis and the citric acid cycle.
- Oxidation of fatty acids to generate energy.

Biological Significance: Exergonic reactions provide the necessary energy for cellular functions such as active transport, biosynthesis, and muscle contraction. They are the main source of energy in metabolism.

b. Endergonic Reactions: Endergonic reactions are reactions that **require an input of energy** to proceed. In these reactions, the free energy of the products is higher than that of the reactants, resulting in a **positive ΔG (ΔG > 0)**. Endergonic reactions are non-spontaneous on their own and must be coupled with exergonic reactions to occur in living cells.

Characteristics of Endergonic Reactions

- ΔG is positive (ΔG > 0).
- Energy must be supplied for the reaction to proceed.
- Reaction is non-spontaneous.
- Often coupled with exergonic reactions (e.g., ATP hydrolysis) to drive the process.

Examples

- Synthesis of glucose from carbon dioxide and water during photosynthesis.
- Formation of peptide bonds during protein synthesis.
- Active transport of ions across cell membranes.

Coupling of Reactions: In biological systems, endergonic reactions are frequently coupled with exergonic reactions, such as ATP hydrolysis. This coupling ensures that the overall ΔG of the combined reaction is negative, allowing energy-requiring processes to occur efficiently.

Relationship between Free Energy, Enthalpy, and Entropy

In biological systems, energy transformations are crucial for sustaining life. The thermodynamic parameters **free energy (G), enthalpy (H), and entropy (S)** provide a quantitative framework to understand these transformations. They are interrelated and collectively determine whether a biochemical reaction is spontaneous, how much work it can perform, and how energy is partitioned between useful work and disorder.

1. Enthalpy (H)

Enthalpy is the **total energy content of a system**, primarily stored in chemical bonds and in the form of heat. It reflects the heat absorbed or released during a reaction at constant pressure.

- **$\Delta H < 0$ (Negative change in enthalpy):** The reaction is exothermic and releases heat to the surroundings. Example: Combustion of glucose or oxidation of nutrients.
- **$\Delta H > 0$ (Positive change in enthalpy):** The reaction is endothermic and absorbs heat from the surroundings. Example: Photosynthesis where energy from sunlight is absorbed to synthesize glucose.

Enthalpy provides information about the energy stored in chemical bonds and the overall energy balance in a reaction.

2. Entropy (S)

Entropy measures the **degree of disorder or randomness** in a system. It is a measure of how energy is dispersed within molecules and the surroundings.

- **$\Delta S > 0$ (Positive change in entropy):** The system becomes more disordered. For instance, the breakdown of glucose into CO_2 and H_2O increases molecular disorder.
- **$\Delta S < 0$ (Negative change in entropy):** The system becomes more ordered. For example, formation of complex macromolecules like proteins or nucleic acids decreases disorder.

Entropy is important in predicting the spontaneity of reactions, especially at different temperatures, because temperature magnifies the effect of ΔS on free energy.

3. Gibbs Free Energy (G)

Gibbs free energy combines enthalpy and entropy into a single value that predicts whether a reaction is **spontaneous** under constant temperature and pressure. The Gibbs free energy change (ΔG) is given by:

$$\Delta G = \Delta H - T\Delta S$$

Where:

- ΔG = Change in Gibbs free energy
- ΔH = Change in enthalpy
- T = Absolute temperature in Kelvin
- ΔS = Change in entropy

Understanding the Equation in Detail

- **ΔH (Enthalpy term):** Reflects the heat energy released or absorbed. Exothermic reactions ($\Delta H < 0$) tend to favor spontaneity because they release energy.
- **$T\Delta S$ (Entropy term):** Reflects the contribution of disorder multiplied by temperature. At higher temperatures, entropy changes have a larger influence on the free energy change.

Predicting Reaction Spontaneity: The signs of ΔH and ΔS determine ΔG and whether a reaction is spontaneous:

1. **$\Delta H < 0$ and $\Delta S > 0$:** ΔG is always negative; reaction is spontaneous at all temperatures (favorable). Example: Cellular respiration.
2. **$\Delta H > 0$ and $\Delta S < 0$:** ΔG is always positive; reaction is non-spontaneous at all temperatures (unfavorable). Example: Formation of complex polymers from simple monomers without energy input.
3. **$\Delta H < 0$ and $\Delta S < 0$:** Reaction may be spontaneous at **low temperatures,** where the enthalpy term dominates. Example: Protein folding in a controlled cellular environment.
4. **$\Delta H > 0$ and $\Delta S > 0$:** Reaction may be spontaneous at **high temperatures**, where the $T\Delta S$ term dominates. Example: Melting of ice or endothermic reactions driven by entropy increase.

Biological Significance of Free Energy Relationship

- **Energy Coupling:** Endergonic reactions ($\Delta G > 0$) that are non-spontaneous can be coupled with exergonic reactions ($\Delta G < 0$) like ATP hydrolysis to drive essential cellular processes.
- **Metabolic Regulation:** Enzymes and metabolic pathways adjust ΔH and ΔS to control the rate and direction of reactions, ensuring

efficiency and homeostasis.

- **Temperature Sensitivity:** Since ΔG depends on temperature, biological systems can exploit temperature changes to regulate processes like enzyme activity and membrane fluidity.
- **Equilibrium Considerations:** When $\Delta G = 0$, the reaction is at equilibrium, meaning no net energy is available for work. Cells constantly shift reactions away from equilibrium using energy inputs to sustain life processes.

Redox Potential (Reduction-Oxidation Potential)

Redox potential, also known as **oxidation-reduction potential (E_0)**, is a measure of the tendency of a chemical species to acquire electrons and undergo reduction. In bioenergetics, redox reactions play a central role in energy transduction, particularly in processes such as **cellular respiration, photosynthesis, and electron transport chains**, where electrons are transferred from electron donors to acceptors, releasing energy in a controlled manner.

Definition of Redox Potential: Redox potential is defined as the **electrical potential difference** of a redox couple, measured in volts (V) or millivolts (mV), relative to a standard reference electrode, usually the **standard hydrogen electrode (SHE)**. It indicates whether a molecule is more likely to **gain electrons (reduction)** or **lose electrons (oxidation)**.

Redox Reactions in Biological Systems: A general redox reaction can be written as:

Oxidized form + e− ↔ Reduced form

- **Oxidized form:** Electron acceptor
- **Reduced form:** Electron donor During such reactions, electrons flow from a molecule with **lower redox potential** (stronger electron donor) to a molecule with **higher redox potential** (stronger electron acceptor).

Standard Redox Potential (E_0'): The **standard redox potential** (E_0') refers to the redox potential measured under standard biochemical conditions:

- pH 7.0
- 25°C (298 K)
- 1 M concentration of reactants and products
- Standard reference electrode (SHE, $E_0 = 0$ V)

A **positive E_0' value** indicates a greater tendency to accept electrons (strong oxidizing agent), while a **negative E_0' value** indicates a greater tendency to donate electrons (strong reducing agent).

Relationship to Free Energy: Redox reactions are closely related to free energy changes in biological systems. The relationship is given by the **Nernst equation**:

$\Delta G = -nF\Delta E$

Where:

- ΔG = Free energy change (J/mol)
- n = Number of electrons transferred
- F = Faraday constant (96,485 C/mol)
- ΔE = Difference in redox potential between electron acceptor and donor (E_0' acceptor – E_0' donor)

A **positive ΔE** corresponds to a negative ΔG, indicating a spontaneous reaction that can release energy for cellular work, such as ATP synthesis.

Biological Examples

- **NAD^+/NADH and FAD/$FADH_2$:** These are key electron carriers in metabolism. NADH has a negative redox potential, making it a strong electron donor, while O_2 has a positive redox potential, making it a strong electron acceptor. Electrons flow spontaneously from NADH to O_2 through the electron transport chain, generating a proton gradient for ATP production.
- **Cytochromes and Iron-Sulfur Proteins:** These proteins act as intermediates in electron transfer, each with specific redox potentials that ensure directional flow of electrons.
- **Photosynthetic Electron Transport:** Electrons move from water (low redox potential) to $NADP^+$ (high redox potential) via photosystems

and carriers, converting light energy into chemical energy.

Significance of Redox Potential in Bioenergetics

- Determines the **direction of electron flow** in metabolic pathways.
- Allows calculation of **energy yield** from oxidation-reduction reactions.
- Explains why certain molecules act as **electron donors** (reducing agents) or **electron acceptors** (oxidizing agents).
- Critical for **cellular energy transduction**, including ATP synthesis and maintenance of membrane potentials.

Energy-Rich Compounds

Energy-rich compounds are molecules that store **high amounts of free energy** in their chemical bonds, which can be readily released to drive biological processes. These compounds play a crucial role in cellular metabolism by providing energy for biosynthesis, active transport, muscle contraction, and other energy-requiring activities. Among these, **adenosine triphosphate (ATP)** is the most well-known and universally used energy currency, but other compounds such as **phosphocreatine, nucleoside triphosphates, and high-energy phosphate intermediates** are also important.

Classification of Energy-Rich Compounds

Energy-rich compounds can be classified based on the **type of high-energy bond** they contain and their **biological roles** in metabolism. These compounds are crucial for energy storage, transfer, and utilization in cells. The classification is generally divided into **phosphate compounds, thioesters, and other high-energy molecules.**

1. Phosphate Compounds

These compounds contain **phosphoanhydride or phosphoester bonds**, which store significant amounts of free energy. The hydrolysis of these bonds releases energy that can drive endergonic reactions.

a) Adenosine Triphosphate (ATP)

- Structure: Adenosine (adenine + ribose) with three phosphate groups.

- High-energy bond: Terminal phosphoanhydride bond.
- Function: Universal energy currency, drives almost all energy-requiring reactions in the cell.

b) Guanosine Triphosphate (GTP)

- Function: Energy donor in protein synthesis (translation), gluconeogenesis, and signal transduction.
- High-energy bond similar to ATP.

c) Uridine Triphosphate (UTP) and Cytidine Triphosphate (CTP)

- UTP: Activates glucose for glycogen synthesis (forms UDP-glucose).
- CTP: Participates in lipid biosynthesis.

d) Phosphocreatine (Creatine Phosphate)

- High-energy phosphate donor, especially in muscle cells.
- Functions as a rapid ATP buffer during short-term high-energy demands.

e) Polyphosphates

- Chains of phosphate units found in some microorganisms.
- Serve as phosphate and energy reservoirs.

2. Thioesters

Thioesters contain a **sulfur atom linked to an acyl group**, forming a high-energy bond. Hydrolysis of thioester bonds releases large amounts of free energy.

a) Acetyl-CoA

- Acetyl group linked to coenzyme A via a thioester bond.
- High-energy bond drives the formation of citrate in the citric acid cycle.
- Serves as a central intermediate in metabolism for energy production and biosynthesis of fatty acids, cholesterol, and ketone bodies.

b) Succinyl-CoA

- Thioester in the citric acid cycle.

- Hydrolysis drives substrate-level phosphorylation, forming GTP/ATP.

3. High-Energy Metabolic Intermediates

Certain intermediates in glycolysis, gluconeogenesis, and other pathways contain high-energy phosphate bonds that can be used for ATP synthesis.

a) 1,3-Bisphosphoglycerate (1,3-BPG)

- Intermediate in glycolysis.
- High phosphoryl transfer potential; donates phosphate to ADP to form ATP.

b) Phosphoenolpyruvate (PEP)

- Glycolytic intermediate with very high free energy of hydrolysis.
- Transfers phosphate to ADP to form ATP via substrate-level phosphorylation.

c) Creatine Phosphate

- Already mentioned under phosphate compounds; serves as immediate energy reserve.

4. Other Energy-Rich Compounds

- **Acyl phosphates**: e.g., acetyl phosphate, propionyl phosphate; involved in certain microbial metabolic pathways.
- **Diphosphate nucleotides**: e.g., ATP, GTP derivatives used in specific biosynthetic reactions.
- **Reduced coenzymes**: NADH, $FADH_2$, and NADPH; although not containing high-energy phosphate bonds, they carry **reducing equivalents** that can be used to generate ATP through oxidative phosphorylation.

Biological Significance of ATP

Adenosine triphosphate (ATP) is universally recognized as the **primary energy currency of the cell**. Its biological significance lies in its ability to store and release energy efficiently to drive virtually all cellular processes that require energy. ATP functions not only as an energy provider but also as a regulator and participant in key metabolic pathways.

1. Immediate Source of Energy

- ATP stores energy in its **phosphoanhydride bonds**, especially the terminal bond. Hydrolysis of ATP to ADP and inorganic phosphate (Pi) releases approximately **30.5 kJ/mol** of free energy under standard conditions.
- This energy is readily available to fuel **cellular activities** such as muscle contraction, nerve impulse propagation, and maintenance of ion gradients.

2. Energy Coupling in Cellular Reactions

- Many biochemical reactions are **endergonic** ($\Delta G > 0$) and cannot occur spontaneously.
- ATP hydrolysis, an **exergonic reaction** ($\Delta G < 0$), is coupled to endergonic reactions to make the overall process spontaneous.
- Examples of coupled processes include:
  - **Biosynthesis of macromolecules:** Formation of proteins, nucleic acids, and polysaccharides.
  - **Active transport:** Pumping ions like Na^+, K^+, and Ca^{2+} against concentration gradients.
  - **Mechanical work:** Muscle contraction and cytoskeletal movements.

3. Substrate-Level Phosphorylation

- ATP can be synthesized directly in metabolic pathways via **substrate-level phosphorylation**, where a high-energy phosphate group from a metabolic intermediate is transferred to ADP.
- Examples:
  - Conversion of 1,3-bisphosphoglycerate to 3-phosphoglycerate in glycolysis.
  - Conversion of phosphoenolpyruvate (PEP) to pyruvate.

4. Role in Signal Transduction

- ATP is a precursor for **cyclic AMP (cAMP)**, an important secondary messenger in cellular signaling.

- cAMP mediates hormonal responses, including regulation of glycogen, lipid, and protein metabolism.
- ATP-dependent phosphorylation of proteins by kinases regulates enzyme activity and signaling pathways.

5. Coenzyme Function

- ATP acts as a **donor of phosphate groups**, adenyl groups, or energy in reactions catalyzed by enzymes.
- In reactions like **amino acid activation** for protein synthesis, ATP provides both the energy and the chemical group required to form high-energy intermediates.

6. Maintenance of Cellular Homeostasis

- ATP provides energy to maintain **ion gradients** across membranes through pumps such as Na^+/K^+-ATPase and Ca^{2+}-ATPase.
- These gradients are essential for processes like nerve impulse transmission, muscle contraction, and nutrient transport.

7. Energy Reservoir and Transfer

- ATP serves as an **energy shuttle**, transferring energy from energy-producing catabolic reactions (e.g., glycolysis, oxidative phosphorylation) to energy-requiring anabolic processes.
- This ensures **efficient energy distribution** without the need to transport heat energy directly.

8. Regulation of Metabolic Pathways

- ATP acts as a **feedback regulator** in many metabolic pathways. High ATP levels inhibit catabolic pathways, whereas low ATP levels stimulate them.
- This regulation helps maintain **energy balance** and prevents excessive accumulation or depletion of metabolites.

Biological Significance of Cyclic AMP (cAMP)

Cyclic adenosine monophosphate (cAMP) is a **secondary messenger** that plays a central role in transducing signals from extracellular stimuli, such as hormones and neurotransmitters, to intracellular targets. It is derived from ATP through the action of the enzyme **adenylate cyclase** and is rapidly degraded by **phosphodiesterase** to regulate its levels. cAMP enables cells to **respond quickly and efficiently** to changes in their environment, making it a key regulator of numerous physiological and biochemical processes.

1. Mediator of Hormonal Action

- cAMP acts as an intracellular messenger for **hormones that bind to G protein-coupled receptors (GPCRs)** on the cell surface.
- Hormones such as **adrenaline, glucagon, and parathyroid hormone** stimulate adenylate cyclase via GPCRs, increasing cAMP levels.
- This leads to activation of **protein kinase A (PKA)**, which phosphorylates target enzymes and proteins, thereby regulating metabolic pathways.
- Example: In liver cells, glucagon increases cAMP, activating enzymes that promote **glycogen breakdown (glycogenolysis)** and **gluconeogenesis**.

2. Regulation of Metabolic Pathways

- cAMP coordinates **energy metabolism** by activating or inhibiting key enzymes through phosphorylation:
    - o **Glycogen metabolism:** Activates glycogen phosphorylase (breakdown) and inhibits glycogen synthase (synthesis).
    - o **Lipid metabolism:** Activates hormone-sensitive lipase, promoting lipolysis in adipose tissue.
    - o **Protein metabolism:** Can regulate proteolytic enzymes in some tissues.

3. Role in Signal Transduction

- cAMP functions as a **secondary messenger**, amplifying signals received by cell-surface receptors.
- A single hormone molecule can generate multiple cAMP molecules, allowing **signal amplification** and a rapid cellular response.

- cAMP mediates cellular responses in many tissues, including heart, liver, adipose tissue, and kidneys.

4. Regulation of Gene Expression

- cAMP can influence transcription by activating **cAMP response element-binding protein (CREB).**
- Phosphorylated CREB binds to specific DNA sequences (cAMP response elements, CRE) in the promoters of target genes.
- This mechanism regulates **long-term changes** in cells, such as differentiation, proliferation, and metabolic enzyme synthesis.

5. Role in Cellular Functions

- **Ion transport:** cAMP regulates ion channels, such as opening chloride channels in epithelial cells (important in intestinal and respiratory secretions).
- **Neurotransmission:** Modulates synaptic activity and neuronal signaling.
- **Cell growth and differentiation:** Influences pathways that control proliferation and differentiation in various cell types.

6. Regulation of Physiological Processes

- **Cardiovascular system:** cAMP mediates the effect of adrenaline on heart rate and contractility.
- **Respiratory system:** Regulates relaxation of smooth muscles in the bronchi via cAMP-mediated pathways.
- **Endocrine system:** Controls hormone secretion and feedback mechanisms.

7. Termination of cAMP Signal

- cAMP levels are tightly regulated by **phosphodiesterase (PDE)**, which hydrolyzes cAMP to AMP, ensuring that the signal is transient and precisely controlled.

Chapter-3

Carbohydrate Metabolism

Carbohydrates are one of the primary macronutrients and serve as a major source of energy for the body. They are organic compounds composed of carbon, hydrogen, and oxygen, generally with the empirical formula Cn(H2O)nC_n(H_2O)_nCn(H2O)n. Carbohydrate metabolism refers to the biochemical processes responsible for the formation, breakdown, and interconversion of carbohydrates in living organisms. These metabolic pathways ensure a continuous supply of energy to maintain cellular functions, support growth, and regulate blood glucose levels.

The metabolism of carbohydrates can be broadly categorized into **catabolic pathways**, which break down carbohydrates to release energy, and **anabolic pathways**, which involve the synthesis of carbohydrates for storage or structural purposes. The catabolic pathways include glycolysis, glycogenolysis, and the citric acid cycle, whereas the anabolic pathways include gluconeogenesis and glycogenesis. Carbohydrate metabolism is tightly regulated by hormonal signals, mainly insulin and glucagon, to maintain homeostasis and provide energy according to the body's needs.

Carbohydrate metabolism also produces intermediates that serve as precursors for the synthesis of nucleotides, amino acids, and lipids. Additionally, it plays a critical role in maintaining blood glucose levels, especially during fasting or intense physical activity, through processes like glycogen breakdown and gluconeogenesis. Dysregulation of carbohydrate metabolism can lead to metabolic disorders such as diabetes mellitus, hypoglycemia, and various glycogen storage diseases, emphasizing its importance in health and disease.

Glycolysis

Glycolysis is the central pathway of carbohydrate catabolism in which one molecule of glucose, a six-carbon sugar, is enzymatically broken down into two molecules of pyruvate, a three-carbon compound. This process occurs in the **cytoplasm** of the cell and does not require oxygen, making it an **anaerobic pathway**. Glycolysis serves as the first step in cellular respiration, providing both energy in the form of ATP and intermediates for other metabolic pathways such as the citric acid cycle and lipid synthesis. Glycolysis is highly conserved across species due to its fundamental role in energy metabolism.

Overview of Glycolysis

Glycolysis involves a series of **ten enzyme-catalyzed reactions** that convert glucose into pyruvate, generating a net gain of energy. It can be divided into two major phases:

1. **Energy Investment Phase (Preparatory Phase):** This phase consumes ATP to phosphorylate glucose and convert it into intermediates that can be split into two three-carbon molecules.
2. **Energy Payoff Phase (Payoff Phase):** This phase generates ATP and NADH by oxidizing the three-carbon intermediates into pyruvate.

Glycolytic Pathway

The glycolytic pathway, also called the **Embden-Meyerhof-Parnas (EMP) pathway**, consists of **ten sequential enzyme-catalyzed reactions** that convert glucose into pyruvate. It can be broadly divided into two phases:

1. **Energy Investment (Preparatory) Phase** – In this phase, the cell consumes energy in the form of ATP to phosphorylate glucose and prepare it for cleavage into two three-carbon molecules. This phase ensures that glucose is chemically activated and trapped inside the cell.
2. **Energy Payoff Phase** – In this phase, the three-carbon intermediates are oxidized and substrate-level phosphorylation occurs, generating ATP and NADH, ultimately yielding pyruvate as the end product.

Stepwise Description of the Glycolytic Pathway

Energy Investment Phase

- **Step 1: Phosphorylation of Glucose**: Glucose is phosphorylated to **glucose-6-phosphate (G6P)** by the enzyme **hexokinase** in most tissues, or **glucokinase** in the liver and pancreatic β-cells. This reaction consumes 1 ATP molecule. Phosphorylation serves two purposes: it **traps glucose inside the cell** and **activates it** for subsequent reactions. Hexokinase is inhibited by its product G6P, while glucokinase has a high Km and is not inhibited by G6P, allowing the liver to regulate blood glucose.
- **Step 2: Isomerization of Glucose-6-Phosphate**: G6P is isomerized to **fructose-6-phosphate (F6P)** by **phosphoglucose isomerase**. This step rearranges the six-carbon aldose (glucose) into a ketose (fructose), facilitating the subsequent phosphorylation and cleavage reactions.
- **Step 3: Phosphorylation of Fructose-6-Phosphate**: F6P is phosphorylated to **fructose-1,6-bisphosphate (F1,6BP)** by **phosphofructokinase-1 (PFK-1)**, consuming another ATP molecule. PFK-1 is the **key rate-limiting enzyme of glycolysis** and is allosterically regulated by cellular energy status: inhibited by ATP and citrate, activated by AMP and fructose-2,6-bisphosphate.
- **Step 4: Cleavage of Fructose-1,6-Bisphosphate**: F1,6BP is split by **aldolase** into two three-carbon sugars: **glyceraldehyde-3-phosphate (G3P)** and **dihydroxyacetone phosphate (DHAP)**. Only G3P continues directly in glycolysis.
- **Step 5: Isomerization of DHAP**: DHAP is converted to G3P by **triose phosphate isomerase**, ensuring that both three-carbon molecules can proceed through the energy payoff phase. At the end of this phase, **two molecules of G3P** are available for subsequent reactions.

Energy Payoff Phase

- **Step 6: Oxidation and Phosphorylation of G3P**: Each G3P molecule is oxidized by **glyceraldehyde-3-phosphate dehydrogenase** to form **1,3-bisphosphoglycerate (1,3-BPG)**. NAD^+ is reduced to **NADH** in this step. 1,3-BPG is a high-energy intermediate capable of transferring its phosphate group to ADP.

- **Step 7: First Substrate-Level Phosphorylation**: 1,3-BPG donates a phosphate group to ADP, forming **ATP** and **3-phosphoglycerate (3-PG)** via **phosphoglycerate kinase**. This is the first ATP-generating step of glycolysis. Since two G3P molecules are formed from one glucose, **two ATP molecules** are generated at this stage.
- **Step 8: Conversion of 3-Phosphoglycerate to 2-Phosphoglycerate**: 3-PG is converted to **2-phosphoglycerate (2-PG)** by **phosphoglycerate mutase**, preparing it for the dehydration step.
- **Step 9: Dehydration of 2-Phosphoglycerate**: 2-PG is dehydrated by **enolase** to form **phosphoenolpyruvate (PEP)**, a high-energy intermediate with a very negative free energy change suitable for ATP synthesis.
- **Step 10: Second Substrate-Level Phosphorylation**: PEP donates its phosphate to ADP, forming **ATP** and **pyruvate** via **pyruvate kinase**. Pyruvate kinase is regulated by ATP (inhibitor), alanine (inhibitor), and fructose-1,6-bisphosphate (activator). Since two PEP molecules are generated per glucose, **two ATP molecules** are produced at this step.

Net Energy Yield per Glucose Molecule

- **ATP:** 4 generated − 2 consumed = **2 ATP (net gain)**
- **NADH:** 2 molecules
- **Pyruvate:** 2 molecules

Energetics of Glycolysis

- Glycolysis is **exergonic overall**, with a negative free energy change, making it energetically favorable.
- The energy investment phase temporarily consumes 2 ATP to prime glucose for breakdown, while the payoff phase generates 4 ATP and 2 NADH.
- NADH produced can enter the **electron transport chain** under

aerobic conditions, leading to additional ATP generation.

- Overall, glycolysis is an efficient mechanism for rapid energy production in the absence or presence of oxygen.

Significance of Glycolysis

1. **Primary Source of ATP:** Glycolysis provides **immediate energy** for cellular functions, particularly in cells lacking mitochondria, such as red blood cells, or in tissues under hypoxic conditions, such as muscle during intense exercise.
2. **Production of Reducing Equivalents:** NADH generated in glycolysis can contribute to **oxidative phosphorylation** in aerobic conditions, increasing overall ATP yield.
3. **Precursor for Biosynthesis:** Intermediates of glycolysis are precursors for essential biomolecules:
   - **3-Phosphoglycerate:** Amino acids like serine, glycine, and cysteine
   - **Dihydroxyacetone phosphate:** Glycerol for triglyceride synthesis
   - **Glucose-6-phosphate:** Pentose phosphate pathway intermediates for nucleotides
4. **Blood Glucose Homeostasis:** Glycolysis regulates the utilization of glucose, indirectly helping maintain **stable blood glucose levels**.
5. **Adaptation to Anaerobic Conditions:** Under low oxygen, pyruvate is converted to **lactate** via lactate dehydrogenase, regenerating NAD^+ for glycolysis and sustaining ATP production.
6. **Integration with Other Pathways:** Glycolysis is closely connected with **gluconeogenesis, glycogen metabolism, and the pentose phosphate pathway**, providing metabolic flexibility and adaptability to varying energy and biosynthetic demands.
7. **Rapid Response:** Glycolysis allows cells to respond quickly to sudden energy demands since it is faster than mitochondrial oxidative phosphorylation.
8. **Evolutionary Significance:** As an ancient metabolic pathway, glycolysis is conserved across species and represents a **fundamental**

energy-yielding mechanism essential for life.

Gluconeogenesis

Gluconeogenesis is the **metabolic process by which glucose is synthesized from non-carbohydrate precursors** such as lactate, glycerol, and glucogenic amino acids. This pathway is essential for maintaining **blood glucose homeostasis**, especially during **fasting, prolonged exercise, starvation, or low-carbohydrate diets**, when dietary glucose is unavailable. Gluconeogenesis primarily occurs in the **liver** and, to a smaller extent, in the **renal cortex**. The pathway ensures a continuous supply of glucose for tissues that are highly dependent on it, such as the **brain, red blood cells, and kidney medulla**. While gluconeogenesis shares many steps with glycolysis, it bypasses the three **irreversible glycolytic reactions** using specific enzymes and energy input to drive the synthesis of glucose.

Precursors for Gluconeogenesis

1. **Lactate:** Produced by anaerobic glycolysis in muscle and red blood cells, lactate is transported to the liver and converted to pyruvate via **lactate dehydrogenase**. This forms the basis of the **Cori cycle**, which recycles lactate back into glucose.

2. **Glycerol:** Derived from the breakdown of triglycerides in adipose tissue. Glycerol is phosphorylated by **glycerol kinase** to form glycerol-3-phosphate, which is then oxidized to **dihydroxyacetone phosphate (DHAP)**, an intermediate of gluconeogenesis.

3. **Glucogenic Amino Acids:** Amino acids such as alanine, glutamine, and aspartate are converted into pyruvate or citric acid cycle intermediates (e.g., oxaloacetate, α-ketoglutarate) that feed into gluconeogenesis.

4. **Propionate:** In ruminants and during odd-chain fatty acid metabolism, propionate is converted into **succinyl-CoA** and subsequently into oxaloacetate, serving as a gluconeogenic substrate.

Stepwise Pathway of Gluconeogenesis

Step 1: Conversion of Pyruvate to Oxaloacetate

- **Enzyme:** Pyruvate carboxylase
- **Location:** Mitochondria
- **Cofactor:** Biotin
- Pyruvate is carboxylated to **oxaloacetate (OAA)** in an ATP-dependent reaction.
- This step **bypasses the irreversible pyruvate kinase step** of glycolysis.
- Oxaloacetate cannot directly cross the mitochondrial membrane, so it is converted to **malate** or **aspartate**, transported to the cytoplasm, and then converted back to oxaloacetate.

Step 2: Conversion of Oxaloacetate to Phosphoenolpyruvate (PEP)

- **Enzyme:** Phosphoenolpyruvate carboxykinase (PEPCK)
- **Location:** Cytoplasm (OAA is transported out as malate/aspartate)
- **Cofactor:** GTP
- OAA undergoes decarboxylation and phosphorylation to form **PEP**, bypassing the irreversible glycolytic pyruvate kinase step.
- PEP is a high-energy intermediate that continues through the gluconeogenic pathway.

Step 3: Reversible Reactions of Glycolysis in Reverse

- PEP is converted to **2-phosphoglycerate,** then to **3-phosphoglycerate**, followed by conversion to **1,3-bisphosphoglycerate** and **glyceraldehyde-3-phosphate (G3P)**.
- These steps use the same enzymes as glycolysis but proceed in reverse due to the relative concentrations of substrates and products.
- **NADH** is consumed in the reduction of 1,3-bisphosphoglycerate to G3P.

Step 4: Formation of Fructose-1,6-Bisphosphate

- G3P and DHAP are combined via **aldolase** to form **fructose-1,6-bisphosphate**.
- This step mirrors the cleavage in glycolysis but in reverse.

Step 5: Conversion of Fructose-1,6-Bisphosphate to Fructose-6-Phosphate

- **Enzyme:** Fructose-1,6-bisphosphatase
- This reaction **bypasses the irreversible phosphofructokinase-1 (PFK-1) step** of glycolysis.
- **Regulation:** Inhibited by AMP and fructose-2,6-bisphosphate; activated by ATP and citrate.

Step 6: Conversion of Fructose-6-Phosphate to Glucose-6-Phosphate

- **Enzyme:** Phosphoglucose isomerase
- A reversible reaction similar to glycolysis.

Step 7: Conversion of Glucose-6-Phosphate to Glucose

- **Enzyme:** Glucose-6-phosphatase
- **Location:** Endoplasmic reticulum of liver and kidney cells
- This step **bypasses the irreversible hexokinase/glucokinase reaction** of glycolysis.
- Free glucose is released into the bloodstream to maintain **blood glucose levels**.

Energy Requirement of Gluconeogenesis

- Gluconeogenesis is energetically demanding:
  - **4 ATP** molecules are used (2 for pyruvate carboxylase and 2 for 3-phosphoglycerate kinase reactions)
  - **2 GTP** molecules are used for PEPCK reactions
  - **2 NADH** molecules are consumed in the reduction of 1,3-bisphosphoglycerate to G3P
- The high energy demand ensures that gluconeogenesis is tightly regulated and occurs only when necessary.

Regulation of Gluconeogenesis

- **Fructose-1,6-bisphosphatase:** Inhibited by AMP and fructose-2,6-bisphosphate; activated by ATP and citrate.
- **Pyruvate carboxylase:** Activated by acetyl-CoA (signals high

energy and availability of precursors).

- Reciprocal regulation with glycolysis ensures that both pathways are not active simultaneously in the same cell, preventing futile cycling.

Significance of Gluconeogenesis

1. **Maintenance of Blood Glucose:** Critical during fasting, starvation, or prolonged exercise, especially for the **brain, red blood cells, and kidney medulla**.
2. **Energy Supply During Exercise:** Lactate produced in muscles is converted back to glucose in the liver via the **Cori cycle**, sustaining energy production in muscles and maintaining glucose homeostasis.
3. **Metabolic Flexibility:** Allows glucose synthesis from **non-carbohydrate sources**, supporting energy metabolism when dietary carbohydrates are scarce.
4. **Prevention of Hypoglycemia:** Ensures adequate glucose levels in the blood, avoiding hypoglycemic conditions that could impair nervous system function.
5. **Integration with Other Pathways:** Connects carbohydrate, lipid, and amino acid metabolism:
   - Glycerol from adipose tissue contributes to glucose synthesis.
   - Amino acids from protein breakdown serve as glucogenic precursors.
   - Lactate from anaerobic glycolysis is recycled into glucose.
6. **Adaptation to Starvation:** During prolonged fasting, glycogen stores are depleted, and gluconeogenesis becomes the **primary source of glucose**.
7. **Supports Biosynthesis:** Intermediates of gluconeogenesis provide substrates for the pentose phosphate pathway and other anabolic reactions.

Citric Acid Cycle (Krebs Cycle or TCA Cycle): The **citric acid cycle (CAC)**, also called the **Krebs cycle** or **tricarboxylic acid (TCA) cycle**, is a key **aerobic metabolic pathway** that takes place in the

mitochondrial matrix of eukaryotic cells. It is central to cellular respiration, serving as the final common pathway for the oxidation of **carbohydrates, fats, and proteins**. The primary purpose of the cycle is to extract **high-energy electrons** from acetyl-CoA in the form of **NADH and $FADH_2$**, which are later used in the **electron transport chain (ETC)** to produce ATP. Additionally, the TCA cycle produces **GTP (or ATP)** and provides intermediates for biosynthesis of amino acids, nucleotides, heme, and fatty acids.

Each molecule of glucose, after glycolysis and oxidative decarboxylation of pyruvate, produces **two molecules of acetyl-CoA**, which enter the TCA cycle. The cycle is **amphibolic**, meaning it functions in both **catabolism** (breaking down molecules for energy) and **anabolism** (providing intermediates for biosynthesis).

Stepwise Pathway of the Citric Acid Cycle

Step 1: Formation of Citrate

- **Enzyme:** Citrate synthase
- **Reaction:** Acetyl-CoA (2C) + Oxaloacetate (4C) → **Citrate (6C)**
- **Mechanism:** Condensation reaction that releases CoA-SH
- **Significance:** This is the **first committed and irreversible step** of the cycle. Citrate is a six-carbon compound that can proceed through the cycle or be exported to the cytoplasm for fatty acid synthesis.

Step 2: Isomerization of Citrate to Isocitrate

- **Enzyme:** Aconitase
- **Reaction:** Citrate → cis-Aconitate → **Isocitrate**
- **Mechanism:** Reversible dehydration-hydration reaction
- **Significance:** The rearrangement moves a hydroxyl group to facilitate subsequent oxidative decarboxylation.

Step 3: Oxidative Decarboxylation of Isocitrate to α-Ketoglutarate

- **Enzyme:** Isocitrate dehydrogenase
- **Reaction:** Isocitrate + NAD^+ → **α-Ketoglutarate (5C) + NADH + CO_2**
- **Significance:** This is the **first oxidative decarboxylation,**

generating NADH and releasing CO_2.

- **Regulation:** Rate-limiting step of the TCA cycle; activated by ADP and Ca^{2+}, inhibited by ATP and NADH.

Step 4: Oxidative Decarboxylation of α-Ketoglutarate to Succinyl-CoA

- **Enzyme:** α-Ketoglutarate dehydrogenase complex
- **Reaction:** α-Ketoglutarate + NAD^+ + CoA → **Succinyl-CoA (4C) + NADH + CO_2**
- **Mechanism:** Similar to pyruvate dehydrogenase, requires **TPP, FAD, NAD^+, CoA, and lipoic acid**
- **Significance:** Second irreversible oxidative decarboxylation; regulated by product inhibition (NADH, Succinyl-CoA) and activated by Ca^{2+}.

Step 5: Conversion of Succinyl-CoA to Succinate

- **Enzyme:** Succinyl-CoA synthetase (succinate thiokinase)
- **Reaction:** Succinyl-CoA + GDP + Pi → **Succinate + GTP + CoA-SH**
- **Mechanism:** Substrate-level phosphorylation generates **GTP**, which can be readily converted to ATP.
- **Significance:** Only substrate-level phosphorylation step in TCA cycle; provides direct energy.

Step 6: Oxidation of Succinate to Fumarate

- **Enzyme:** Succinate dehydrogenase
- **Reaction:** Succinate + FAD → **Fumarate + $FADH_2$**
- **Significance:** Generates $FADH_2$, which donates electrons directly to the **electron transport chain (Complex II)**. Succinate dehydrogenase is **membrane-bound**, linking TCA with oxidative phosphorylation.

Step 7: Hydration of Fumarate to Malate

- **Enzyme:** Fumarase (fumarate hydratase)
- **Reaction:** Fumarate + H_2O → **Malate**
- **Significance:** Prepares malate for final oxidation to oxaloacetate.

Step 8: Oxidation of Malate to Oxaloacetate

- **Enzyme:** Malate dehydrogenase
- **Reaction:** Malate + NAD^+ → **Oxaloacetate + NADH + H^+**
- **Significance:** Regenerates oxaloacetate to condense with a new acetyl-CoA, completing the cycle.

Energetics of the Citric Acid Cycle (per acetyl-CoA molecule)

- **3 NADH → ~7.5 ATP** (via oxidative phosphorylation)
- **1 $FADH_2$ → ~1.5 ATP**
- **1 GTP → 1 ATP** (substrate-level phosphorylation)
- **Total ATP per acetyl-CoA:** ~10 ATP
- **Total ATP per glucose (2 acetyl-CoA):** ~20 ATP from TCA alone, in addition to glycolysis and pyruvate dehydrogenase contributions (~4 ATP via glycolysis and 5 ATP via pyruvate decarboxylation).

Significance of the Citric Acid Cycle

1. **Energy Production:** The primary source of **high-energy electrons (NADH, $FADH_2$)** for the electron transport chain, which produces the majority of cellular ATP under aerobic conditions.
2. **Carbon Dioxide Formation:** Two molecules of CO_2 are released per acetyl-CoA, representing **complete oxidation of carbon atoms**.
3. **Source of Biosynthetic Intermediates:** Intermediates serve as precursors for multiple anabolic pathways:
    - **Citrate:** Exported for **fatty acid and cholesterol synthesis**
    - **α-Ketoglutarate:** Used for **glutamate and other amino acids**
    - **Succinyl-CoA:** Precursor for **heme synthesis**
    - **Oxaloacetate:** Precursor for **aspartate and gluconeogenesis**
4. **Metabolic Integration:** Links **carbohydrate, lipid, and protein metabolism**. Acetyl-CoA can be derived from pyruvate, fatty acids, or amino acids, making the TCA cycle a metabolic hub.
5. **Regulation of Cellular Metabolism:** The cycle is tightly regulated at **citrate synthase, isocitrate dehydrogenase, and α-ketoglutarate dehydrogenase**, responsive to ATP, ADP, NADH, and

Ca^{2+} levels, ensuring energy balance.

6. **Support for Aerobic Respiration:** Provides reducing equivalents (NADH, $FADH_2$) for oxidative phosphorylation, which generates the **majority of ATP in aerobic cells**.

7. **Adaptation to Nutritional Status:** During fasting, acetyl-CoA from fatty acid oxidation enters the cycle for energy, while intermediates may be withdrawn for **gluconeogenesis and amino acid synthesis**, highlighting its amphibolic nature.

8. **Detoxification and Nitrogen Metabolism:** Provides carbon skeletons for **urea cycle** and supports detoxification of nitrogenous compounds.

Hexose Monophosphate (HMP) Shunt

The **Hexose Monophosphate (HMP) Shunt**, also called the **Pentose Phosphate Pathway (PPP)**, is an alternative metabolic pathway for **glucose oxidation**, distinct from glycolysis. Unlike glycolysis, which primarily generates ATP, the HMP shunt serves **biosynthetic and antioxidant functions** by producing **NADPH** and **pentose sugars** (5-carbon sugars). This pathway occurs entirely in the **cytosol** of cells and is particularly active in tissues with **high biosynthetic activity** such as the **liver, adipose tissue, adrenal cortex, mammary glands**, and in **red blood cells**, where it helps maintain **reduced glutathione (GSH)** to protect against oxidative damage.

The HMP shunt is an **amphibolic pathway**, providing both reducing power and metabolic intermediates. It operates in coordination with glycolysis, adjusting to the cellular requirements for NADPH, ribose-5-phosphate, and energy.

Objectives of the HMP Shunt

1. **Generation of NADPH** for reductive biosynthesis and detoxification reactions.

2. **Production of ribose-5-phosphate** for nucleotide and nucleic acid synthesis.

3. **Interconversion of sugars** to support glycolysis, gluconeogenesis, or biosynthetic demands.

4. **Protection against oxidative stress** by maintaining reduced glutathione.

Precursors and Substrates

- **Primary substrate:** Glucose-6-phosphate (derived from glucose via hexokinase/glucokinase)
- **Coenzymes:** $NADP^+$ (oxidized form, reduced to NADPH)
- **Products:** NADPH, CO_2, ribulose-5-phosphate, and sugar intermediates that can enter glycolysis

Phases of the HMP Shunt

The HMP shunt consists of **two interconnected phases**:

1. Oxidative Phase (Irreversible Reactions)

This phase generates **NADPH** and produces **ribulose-5-phosphate.**

Step 1: Oxidation of Glucose-6-Phosphate

- **Enzyme:** Glucose-6-phosphate dehydrogenase (G6PD)
- **Reaction:** Glucose-6-phosphate + $NADP^+$ → **6-phosphoglucono-δ-lactone + NADPH + H^+**
- **Significance:**
  - Rate-limiting and regulatory step of the HMP shunt.
  - Activated by $NADP^+$ (indicating need for reducing equivalents).
  - Inhibited by high NADPH levels.

Step 2: Hydrolysis of 6-Phosphoglucono-δ-Lactone

- **Enzyme:** Lactonase (6-phosphogluconolactonase)
- **Reaction:** 6-Phosphoglucono-δ-lactone + H_2O → **6-Phosphogluconate**
- Converts the lactone to an open-chain form suitable for decarboxylation.

Step 3: Oxidative Decarboxylation of 6-Phosphogluconate

- **Enzyme:** 6-Phosphogluconate dehydrogenase
- **Reaction:** 6-Phosphogluconate + $NADP^+$ → **Ribulose-5-phosphate + NADPH + CO_2**

- Produces a **second molecule of NADPH** per glucose-6-phosphate.
- Releases CO_2, representing the first loss of a carbon from glucose.

Outcome of Oxidative Phase

- 2 molecules of NADPH generated per glucose-6-phosphate
- 1 molecule of ribulose-5-phosphate produced

2. Non-Oxidative Phase (Reversible Sugar Interconversions)

This phase interconverts **pentose sugars** to produce **ribose-5-phosphate** for nucleotide synthesis or **glycolytic intermediates** (fructose-6-phosphate and glyceraldehyde-3-phosphate) depending on cellular needs.

Step 1: Isomerization and Epimerization

- **Ribulose-5-phosphate** → **Ribose-5-phosphate** (via phosphopentose isomerase)
  - Ribose-5-phosphate is used for **nucleotide and nucleic acid synthesis.**
- **Ribulose-5-phosphate** → **Xylulose-5-phosphate** (via phosphopentose epimerase)

Step 2: Carbon Skeleton Rearrangement (Transketolase and Transaldolase Reactions)

- **Transketolase:** Transfers 2-carbon units between sugars (requires **TPP, thiamine pyrophosphate**)
  - Example: Xylulose-5-phosphate + Ribose-5-phosphate → Glyceraldehyde-3-phosphate + Sedoheptulose-7-phosphate
- **Transaldolase:** Transfers 3-carbon units between sugars
  - Example: Sedoheptulose-7-phosphate + Glyceraldehyde-3-phosphate → Erythrose-4-phosphate + Fructose-6-phosphate
- These reactions allow the **recycling of pentoses into hexoses and trioses**, which can enter glycolysis or gluconeogenesis.

Significance of Non-Oxidative Phase

- Produces **ribose-5-phosphate** for nucleotide synthesis.
- Generates **glycolytic intermediates** for energy production or further biosynthetic reactions.

- Balances cellular demand between **NADPH production and ribose sugar synthesis**.

Energetics of the HMP Shunt

- Direct ATP production is **absent**.
- NADPH generated is a **high-energy electron donor** for reductive biosynthesis and antioxidant defense.
- Carbon atoms can be redirected into glycolysis intermediates for **ATP production** if energy is needed.

Regulation of the HMP Shunt

1. **Glucose-6-Phosphate Dehydrogenase (G6PD)**
   - Activated by **NADP⁺** (when NADPH demand is high)
   - Inhibited by **NADPH** (feedback inhibition)
2. **Transketolase**
   - Requires **thiamine pyrophosphate (TPP)**; thiamine deficiency reduces non-oxidative reactions.
3. **Substrate Availability**
   - Abundant glucose-6-phosphate promotes flux through the pathway.

Significance of the HMP Shunt

1. **NADPH Production**
   - Provides reducing equivalents for:
     - **Fatty acid synthesis** in liver, adipose tissue, mammary glands
     - **Cholesterol and steroid hormone synthesis** in adrenal cortex and gonads
     - **Cytochrome P450-mediated detoxification** in liver
     - **Maintenance of reduced glutathione (GSH)** in red blood cells to neutralize reactive oxygen species
2. **Ribose-5-Phosphate Production**
   - Essential for **nucleotide and nucleic acid synthesis** (DNA, RNA, ATP, NADH, FAD, CoA)
   - Critical for **rapidly dividing cells** (bone marrow, skin, cancer cells)

3. Integration with Glycolysis

o Produces **fructose-6-phosphate and glyceraldehyde-3-phosphate**, which can enter glycolysis or gluconeogenesis depending on cellular energy requirements.

4. Antioxidant Defense

o NADPH keeps **glutathione reduced**, protecting red blood cells from oxidative damage.

o G6PD deficiency leads to **hemolytic anemia** under oxidative stress.

5. Support for Biosynthesis

o Supplies NADPH for anabolic reactions including **fatty acid and cholesterol synthesis**, steroid hormone production, and detoxification reactions.

6. Metabolic Flexibility

o Allows the cell to **balance production of NADPH, ribose sugars, and energy**, depending on immediate needs.

Glucose-6-Phosphate Dehydrogenase (G6PD) Deficiency

Glucose-6-phosphate dehydrogenase (G6PD) deficiency is a **hereditary enzymatic disorder** affecting the **Hexose Monophosphate (HMP) shunt** in red blood cells (RBCs). G6PD is the **first and rate-limiting enzyme** in the oxidative phase of the HMP shunt, converting **glucose-6-phosphate to 6-phosphoglucono-δ-lactone**, while generating **NADPH**.

NADPH is critical in RBCs because it maintains **glutathione in its reduced form (GSH)**. Reduced glutathione detoxifies **reactive oxygen species (ROS)**, protecting hemoglobin and the RBC membrane from oxidative damage. RBCs, lacking mitochondria, rely **entirely on the HMP shunt** for NADPH production. Therefore, G6PD deficiency leads to **susceptibility to oxidative stress**, resulting in **hemolysis**.

G6PD deficiency is one of the **most common enzyme deficiencies worldwide**, with high prevalence in **malaria-endemic regions,** reflecting a protective evolutionary effect against malaria.

Genetic Basis and Inheritance

- **Gene Location:** X chromosome (Xq28)
- **Inheritance Pattern:** X-linked recessive
  - **Males:** Hemizygous; usually affected
  - **Females:** Heterozygous; may be carriers or have variable expression due to **X-chromosome inactivation (lyonization)**
- **Molecular Defect:** Missense mutations leading to:
  - Reduced **enzyme activity**
  - Decreased **enzyme stability**
  - Altered **binding to NADP$^+$ or substrate**

Pathophysiology

1. **Defective NADPH Production**
   - G6PD deficiency impairs the oxidative phase of HMP shunt.
   - RBCs cannot produce sufficient **NADPH**, which is needed to reduce **oxidized glutathione (GSSG) to GSH**.
2. **Accumulation of Reactive Oxygen Species (ROS)**
   - Without adequate GSH, ROS accumulate, oxidizing hemoglobin and membrane lipids.
3. **Formation of Heinz Bodies**
   - Oxidized hemoglobin precipitates within RBCs, forming **Heinz bodies**, which are visible on supravital staining.
4. **RBC Membrane Damage**
   - Lipid peroxidation weakens the membrane, making RBCs **fragile and prone to hemolysis** in the spleen.
5. **Hemolysis**
   - Can be **acute**, triggered by oxidative stress, or **chronic** in severe enzyme deficiency.
   - Hemolysis leads to **anemia, jaundice, and hemoglobinuria**.

Triggers of Hemolysis

- **Drugs**
  - Antimalarials: **Primaquine, Chloroquine**

- Sulfonamides: **Sulfamethoxazole, Sulfadiazine**
- Nitrofurantoin
- Dapsone
- High-dose aspirin

- **Foods:** Fava beans (favism)
- **Infections:** Bacterial or viral infections produce oxidative stress
- **Chemicals:** Naphthalene (mothballs), certain dyes

Clinical Manifestations

1. **Acute Hemolytic Anemia**

- Triggered by drugs, fava beans, or infection
- Symptoms: Fatigue, pallor, jaundice, dark urine (hemoglobinuria), back pain
- Onset: Usually **24–72 hours after exposure**

2. **Neonatal Jaundice**

- Excessive bilirubin in newborns
- Severe cases can lead to **kernicterus** if untreated

3. **Chronic Nonspherocytic Hemolytic Anemia (CNSHA)**

- Rare, severe form
- Continuous mild anemia without significant oxidative triggers
- Associated with Class I mutations

Laboratory Findings

- **Peripheral Blood Smear**
    - **Heinz bodies** (denatured hemoglobin)
    - **Bite cells** due to splenic removal of Heinz bodies
- **Complete Blood Count (CBC)**
    - Normocytic, normochromic anemia
    - Reticulocytosis as compensatory response
- **Biochemical Tests**
    - Reduced **G6PD enzyme activity** in RBCs (definitive diagnosis)
    - Indirect hyperbilirubinemia during hemolytic episodes
- **Urine**
    - Hemoglobinuria during acute hemolytic attacks

Classification of G6PD Deficiency (WHO)

Class	Enzyme Activity	Clinical Manifestation
I	<10%	Chronic nonspherocytic hemolytic anemia (CNSHA)
II	<10%	Acute hemolytic anemia
III	10–60%	Usually asymptomatic; hemolysis under oxidative stress
IV	60–100%	Normal; no clinical symptoms
V	>100%	Rare; no clinical significance

Pathophysiological Sequence During Hemolysis

1. Exposure to oxidative stress
2. Increased ROS in RBCs
3. Oxidation of hemoglobin → Heinz bodies formation
4. Damage to RBC membrane → Membrane rigidity and loss
5. Splenic sequestration and destruction → Hemolytic anemia
6. Release of hemoglobin → Indirect hyperbilirubinemia and hemoglobinuria
7. Bone marrow compensates → Reticulocytosis

Management

1. **Avoidance of Triggers**
   - Known drugs, fava beans, chemicals, and infections should be avoided whenever possible.
2. **Treatment of Acute Hemolytic Episodes**
   - Supportive care: Hydration, oxygen therapy
   - Blood transfusion in severe anemia
   - Treat underlying infections if present
3. **Prevention and Counseling**
   - Genetic counseling for affected families

- o Screening in populations with high prevalence

Significance

1. **Clinical Significance**
   - o Most common cause of **drug-induced hemolytic anemia**
   - o Important in **neonatal hyperbilirubinemia,** with risk of **kernicterus**
2. **Evolutionary Significance**
   - o G6PD deficiency confers **partial protection against malaria** (especially Plasmodium falciparum), explaining high prevalence in endemic regions
3. **Metabolic Significance**
   - o Demonstrates the **critical role of the HMP shunt** in RBCs
   - o Highlights the importance of **NADPH and glutathione** in oxidative stress defense
4. **Biochemical Significance**
   - o Links enzyme deficiency to clinical hemolytic episodes
   - o Shows **interdependence between metabolic pathways (HMP shunt) and redox homeostasis**

Glycogen Metabolism

Glycogen is a highly branched polymer of glucose, composed of **α-1,4-linked glucose chains** with **α-1,6-linked branches** approximately every 8–12 glucose units. It serves as the **major storage form of glucose in animals**, primarily in the **liver (10% of liver weight)** and **skeletal muscles (1–2% of muscle weight)**. Liver glycogen maintains **blood glucose levels** during fasting, while muscle glycogen supplies **energy for muscle contraction** during exercise.

Glycogen metabolism is a **dynamic, tightly regulated process**, involving **glycogenesis (synthesis)** and **glycogenolysis (breakdown)**, which are reciprocally regulated to prevent a futile cycle. Hormonal and allosteric regulation ensures metabolic flexibility according to **nutritional and physiological states**.

1. Glycogenesis (Glycogen Synthesis)

Objective: Conversion of glucose into glycogen for **energy storage** when glucose availability is high (fed state).

Stepwise Pathway

Step 1: Glucose Uptake and Phosphorylation

- **Enzymes:**
  - **Hexokinase (muscle)** – low Km, active at physiological glucose levels
  - **Glucokinase (liver)** – high Km, active when glucose is abundant
- **Reaction:** Glucose + ATP → **Glucose-6-phosphate (G6P)**
- **Significance:** Traps glucose inside cells and channels it toward glycogen synthesis

Step 2: Conversion of G6P to Glucose-1-Phosphate (G1P)

- **Enzyme:** Phosphoglucomutase
- **Reaction:** Glucose-6-phosphate ⇌ **Glucose-1-phosphate**
- **Mechanism:** A phosphoryl group is transferred from **C1 to C6** via a **glucose-1,6-bisphosphate intermediate**

Step 3: Formation of UDP-Glucose (Activated Glucose)

- **Enzyme:** UDP-glucose pyrophosphorylase
- **Reaction:** G1P + UTP → **UDP-glucose + PPi**
- **Significance:** UDP-glucose acts as an **activated donor of glucose residues** for glycogen elongation

Step 4: Glycogen Chain Elongation

- **Enzyme:** Glycogen synthase (rate-limiting enzyme of glycogenesis)
- **Reaction:** UDP-glucose + Glycogen(n) → Glycogen(n+1) + UDP
- **Linkage:** Forms **α-1,4-glycosidic bonds**
- **Regulation:**
  - **Activated by:** Glucose-6-phosphate, insulin (via dephosphorylation)
  - **Inhibited by:** Glucagon and epinephrine (via phosphorylation)

Step 5: Formation of Branch Points

- **Enzyme:** Glycogen branching enzyme (amylo-(1,4→1,6)-transglycosylase)
- **Reaction:** Transfers ~7 glucose residues from the end of a chain to form an ***α*-1,6 branch**
- **Significance:**
  - Increases glycogen **solubility**
  - Creates more **non-reducing ends** for rapid glycogen breakdown
  - Enhances **storage efficiency**

Regulation of Glycogenesis

- **Hormonal Regulation:**
  - **Insulin:** Activates glycogen synthase via **dephosphorylation** (via protein phosphatase-1)
  - **Glucagon / Epinephrine:** Inhibit glycogen synthase via **cAMP-dependent phosphorylation**
- **Allosteric Regulation:**
  - **Glucose-6-phosphate:** Activates glycogen synthase
  - **ATP / citrate:** Indirectly favor glycogenesis

2. Glycogenolysis (Glycogen Breakdown)

Objective: Mobilization of glycogen to release glucose during **fasting, exercise, or stress**.

Stepwise Pathway

Step 1: Phosphorolysis of Glycogen

- **Enzyme:** Glycogen phosphorylase (rate-limiting enzyme)
- **Reaction:** Glycogen(n) + Pi → **Glucose-1-phosphate + Glycogen(n-1)**
- **Mechanism:** Cleaves **α-1,4-glycosidic bonds** at the **non-reducing ends** using inorganic phosphate
- **Significance:** Produces G1P without consuming ATP

Step 2: Debranching of Glycogen

- **Enzyme:** Glycogen debranching enzyme (bifunctional enzyme)

1. **4-α-D-glucanotransferase (transferase activity):** Transfers three glucose residues near the branch point to a nearby chain
2. **Amylo-α-1,6-glucosidase (glucosidase activity):** Hydrolyzes the α-1,6 linkage at branch points to release **free glucose**

Step 3: Conversion of G1P to G6P

- **Enzyme:** Phosphoglucomutase
- **Reaction:** Glucose-1-phosphate ⇌ **Glucose-6-phosphate**

Step 4: Release of Free Glucose (Liver and Kidney Specific)

- **Enzyme:** Glucose-6-phosphatase
- **Reaction:** Glucose-6-phosphate → **Glucose + Pi**
- **Significance:** Provides **glucose for blood circulation**, maintaining normoglycemia during fasting
- **Note:** Muscle lacks glucose-6-phosphatase; G6P enters **glycolysis for ATP production**

Regulation of Glycogenolysis

- **Hormonal Regulation:**
  - **Glucagon (liver) / Epinephrine (liver & muscle):** Activate glycogen phosphorylase via **cAMP-dependent phosphorylation**
  - **Insulin:** Inhibits glycogen phosphorylase via **dephosphorylation**
- **Allosteric Regulation:**
  - **ATP / Glucose-6-phosphate:** Inhibit glycogen phosphorylase
  - **AMP:** Activates glycogen phosphorylase (muscle-specific)

Glycogen Storage Diseases (GSD)

Glycogen Storage Diseases (GSDs) are a group of **inherited metabolic disorders** characterized by **abnormal glycogen metabolism**, resulting in **accumulation of glycogen** in tissues or **deficiency in glycogen mobilization**. These disorders arise due to **defective enzymes involved in glycogenesis or glycogenolysis**, leading to **abnormal glycogen structure or quantity**.

GSDs are typically classified based on the **enzyme defect, affected tissue (liver, muscle, or both), and clinical presentation**. Most GSDs are **autosomal recessive**, except for **Andersen disease (GSD IV)** and some **X-linked forms**. Clinical manifestations include **hepatomegaly, hypoglycemia, growth retardation, and muscle weakness**.

Classification of GSDs

GSDs are classified by **enzyme defect, gene, tissue involved, and clinical features**. The **classical types (I–IX)** are widely recognized:

Type	Name	Enzyme Defect	Tissue Affected	Key Clinical Features
I	Von Gierke disease	Glucose-6-phosphatase	Liver, kidney	Severe fasting **hypoglycemia, hepatomegaly, lactic acidosis, hyperuricemia, hyperlipidemia**
II	Pompe disease	Lysosomal α-1,4-glucosidase (acid maltase)	Muscle, heart, liver	**Cardiomegaly**, hypotonia, **muscle weakness**, early death in infants (classic form)
III	Cori / Forbes disease	Debranching enzyme (α-1,6-glucosidase)	Liver, muscle	**Hepatomegaly**, mild hypoglycemia, muscle weakness
IV	Andersen disease	Branching enzyme (amylo-(1,4→1,6)-transglycosylase)	Liver, spleen	Hepatomegaly, cirrhosis, failure to

				thrive, rare survival
V	McArdle disease	Muscle glycogen phosphorylase	Muscle	Exercise-induced **muscle cramps**, fatigue, **myoglobinuria**
VI	Hers disease	Liver glycogen phosphorylase	Liver	Hepatomegaly, mild hypoglycemia
VII	Tarui disease	Muscle phosphofructokinase	Muscle	Exercise intolerance, muscle cramps, hemolysis
IX	Phosphorylase kinase deficiency	Phosphorylase kinase	Liver / Muscle	Hepatomegaly, growth retardation, mild hypoglycemia

Pathophysiology

1. **Enzyme Deficiency**

o Defective enzymes in glycogen synthesis or breakdown lead to **impaired glucose storage or mobilization**.

2. **Glycogen Accumulation or Abnormal Structure**

o Abnormal glycogen accumulates in **liver, muscle, heart, or kidney**, causing **organomegaly** and **functional impairment**.

o Some forms have **abnormal branching or amylopectin-like glycogen**, e.g., Andersen disease (GSD IV).

3. **Hypoglycemia**

- o Liver GSDs (I, III, VI, IX) → impaired glycogenolysis → **fasting hypoglycemia**
- o Muscle GSDs (V, VII) → exercise intolerance, inability to mobilize glycogen for ATP production

4. **Secondary Metabolic Effects**

- o **Hyperuricemia** and **lactic acidosis** due to shunting of glucose to alternative pathways (GSD I)
- o Lipid abnormalities due to **increased gluconeogenesis and fat metabolism**

Clinical Features

Liver Involvement

- **Hepatomegaly**: Enlarged liver due to glycogen accumulation
- **Hypoglycemia**: Especially during fasting
- **Growth retardation**: Short stature due to chronic hypoglycemia
- **Metabolic abnormalities**: Hyperlactatemia, hyperlipidemia, hyperuricemia

Muscle Involvement

- **Exercise intolerance**: Muscle fatigues quickly during activity
- **Cramps and stiffness**: Due to inability to utilize glycogen
- **Myoglobinuria**: Dark urine after intense exercise (McArdle disease)
- **Cardiomyopathy**: Seen in Pompe disease due to glycogen accumulation in the heart

Other Systemic Features

- Failure to thrive in infancy (severe forms)
- Cirrhosis and liver failure in Andersen disease
- Rare neurological involvement in some forms

Diagnosis

1. **Clinical Evaluation**

- o History of **fasting hypoglycemia, hepatomegaly, muscle cramps, exercise intolerance**

- o Family history for **inheritance pattern**

2. **Laboratory Tests**

- o **Blood glucose:** Low during fasting
- o **Lactate, uric acid, triglycerides:** Often elevated
- o **Creatine kinase (CK):** Elevated in muscle GSDs
- o **Urine:** Myoglobinuria in McArdle disease

3. **Enzyme Assays**

- o Measure specific enzyme activity in **liver biopsy, muscle biopsy, or leukocytes**

4. **Molecular Genetic Testing**

- o Confirms mutation in the gene encoding the defective enzyme

5. **Imaging**

- o Ultrasound or MRI shows **hepatomegaly or muscle glycogen accumulation**

Management

General Principles

- Supportive and symptomatic treatment
- Avoid triggers of hypoglycemia or muscle stress

Liver GSDs (I, III, VI, IX)

- Frequent **small meals, cornstarch therapy** for sustained glucose
- Monitor **growth and metabolic parameters**
- Liver transplant in severe cirrhosis (rare)

Muscle GSDs (V, VII)

- **Moderate exercise** to improve tolerance
- Avoid strenuous activity that triggers **cramps or rhabdomyolysis**
- High-protein diet may be beneficial

Pompe Disease (GSD II)

- **Enzyme replacement therapy (ERT)** with recombinant acid α-glucosidase
- Supportive cardiac and respiratory care

Significance

1. **Metabolic Insight**

- Demonstrates importance of **glycogen metabolism in energy homeostasis**
- Highlights the **role of specific enzymes** in different tissues

2. **Clinical Relevance**
   - Early recognition prevents **hypoglycemia, growth retardation, and organ damage**
   - Guides **dietary and enzyme-based therapy**
3. **Genetic Counseling**
   - Most GSDs are **autosomal recessive** → family planning considerations

Hormonal Regulation of Blood Glucose Level

Blood glucose levels are tightly regulated within a **narrow range (approximately 70–110 mg/dL)** to ensure a **constant supply of glucose** for organs, especially the **brain, red blood cells, and renal medulla**, which rely heavily on glucose. This regulation is achieved by a **complex interplay of hormones** that **increase or decrease blood glucose** in response to **feeding, fasting, exercise, or stress**. The major hormones involved are **insulin, glucagon, epinephrine, cortisol, and growth hormone**, with additional minor contributions from **thyroid hormones**.

1. Insulin – Hypoglycemic Hormone

Source: β-cells of **pancreatic islets of Langerhans**

Stimuli for Secretion

- High blood glucose (postprandial)
- Elevated amino acids (arginine, leucine)
- Gastrointestinal hormones (**incretins** like GLP-1 and GIP)

Target Tissues: Liver, skeletal muscle, adipose tissue

Mechanism of Action

- Insulin binds to **tyrosine kinase receptors**, activating signaling pathways that:

1. **Promote glucose uptake** via **GLUT4 transporters** in muscle and adipose tissue

2. **Stimulate glycogenesis** (glycogen synthesis)
3. **Activate glycolysis** for energy production
4. **Promote lipogenesis** in adipose tissue
5. **Enhance protein synthesis** in muscle

Effect on Blood Glucose

- **Lowers blood glucose** by facilitating glucose storage and utilization
- Inhibits **gluconeogenesis** and **glycogenolysis** in the liver

2. Glucagon – Hyperglycemic Hormone

Source: α-cells of **pancreatic islets of Langerhans**

Stimuli for Secretion

- Low blood glucose (hypoglycemia)
- High amino acids (arginine)
- Exercise-induced stress

Target Tissue: Primarily the **liver**

Mechanism of Action

- Glucagon binds to **G-protein coupled receptors,** activating **adenylate cyclase → cAMP → PKA pathway**
- Effects in the liver:

1. **Stimulates glycogenolysis** → glucose-1-phosphate → glucose
2. **Activates gluconeogenesis** → synthesis of glucose from amino acids and lactate
3. **Inhibits glycogenesis** → prevents storage during fasting

Effect on Blood Glucose

- **Raises blood glucose** by mobilizing glycogen and promoting glucose synthesis

3. Epinephrine – Stress Hormone

Source: Adrenal medulla

Stimuli for Secretion

- Physical stress, exercise, hypoglycemia
- Sympathetic nervous system activation

Target Tissues: Liver, muscle, adipose tissue

Mechanism of Action

- Epinephrine binds to **β-adrenergic receptors**, activating **cAMP-PKA pathway**
- Effects:

1. **Glycogenolysis in liver and muscle** → rapid glucose release
2. **Lipolysis in adipose tissue** → free fatty acids as alternative energy
3. **Inhibition of insulin release** from pancreatic β-cells

Effect on Blood Glucose

- **Rapid increase** in blood glucose during stress or exercise to meet energy demands

4. Cortisol – Glucocorticoid Hormone

Source: Adrenal cortex

Stimuli for Secretion

- Stress (physical or psychological)
- Circadian rhythm (highest in early morning)

Target Tissues: Liver, muscle, adipose tissue

Mechanism of Action

- Cortisol binds to **intracellular glucocorticoid receptors** → alters **gene transcription**
- Effects:

1. **Stimulates gluconeogenesis** in the liver
2. **Inhibits peripheral glucose uptake** (muscle and adipose tissue)
3. **Promotes protein catabolism** → amino acids for gluconeogenesis
4. **Enhances lipolysis** → glycerol for gluconeogenesis

Effect on Blood Glucose

- **Raises blood glucose** during prolonged stress or fasting
- Contributes to **hyperglycemia in Cushing's syndrome**

5. Growth Hormone (GH) – Anti-Insulin Hormone

Source: Anterior pituitary

Stimuli for Secretion

- Hypoglycemia

- Exercise, stress, sleep

Target Tissues: Liver, muscle, adipose tissue

Mechanism of Action

- GH promotes **lipolysis**, reduces **glucose uptake by muscle and adipose tissue**, and **stimulates hepatic gluconeogenesis**
- Indirect effects via **IGF-1 (insulin-like growth factor-1)** contribute to growth

Effect on Blood Glucose

- **Raises blood glucose** by decreasing peripheral glucose utilization and increasing hepatic glucose production

6. Minor Contributors

Thyroid Hormones (T3/T4)

- Enhance **glucose absorption** in the intestine and **gluconeogenesis**
- Moderate hyperglycemic effect

Incretins (GLP-1, GIP)

- Enhance **insulin secretion** postprandially
- Suppress glucagon release

Hormonal Regulation during Different Physiological States

State	Primary Hormones Active	Mechanism	Effect on Blood Glucose
Fed / Postprandial	Insulin ↑	Glucose uptake, glycogenesis, glycolysis	↓ Blood glucose
Fasting / Early Starvation	Glucagon ↑, Cortisol ↑	Glycogenolysis, gluconeogenesis	↑ Blood glucose
Exercise / Stress	Epinephrine ↑, GH ↑, Cortisol ↑	Glycogenolysis, gluconeogenesis, lipolysis	↑ Blood glucose

Prolonged Starvation	Cortisol ↑, GH ↑	Gluconeogenesis, protein catabolism	↑ Blood glucose

Integration and Balance

- **Insulin and glucagon** act as the **primary regulators**, maintaining blood glucose in a **narrow physiological range**.
- **Counter-regulatory hormones** (epinephrine, cortisol, GH) prevent **hypoglycemia** during **stress, fasting, or exercise**.
- **Insulin dominance:** promotes **storage of nutrients** (glycogenesis, lipogenesis, protein synthesis).
- **Glucagon / counter-regulatory hormone dominance:** promotes **mobilization of glucose** (glycogenolysis, gluconeogenesis, lipolysis).

Diabetes Mellitus

Diabetes mellitus is a **chronic metabolic disorder** characterized by **persistent hyperglycemia** resulting from **defects in insulin secretion, insulin action, or both**. Insulin is a key hormone required for the regulation of **carbohydrate, lipid, and protein metabolism**, and its deficiency or ineffectiveness leads to widespread metabolic disturbances. Diabetes mellitus is a major global health problem and is associated with **acute metabolic complications** as well as **long-term damage to multiple organs**, particularly the **eyes, kidneys, nerves, heart, and blood vessels**.

Definition: Diabetes mellitus may be defined as a **group of metabolic diseases** characterized by **chronic hyperglycemia** due to impaired **insulin secretion, insulin action, or both**, accompanied by disturbances in **carbohydrate, fat, and protein metabolism**.

Classification of Diabetes Mellitus

1. Type 1 Diabetes Mellitus (Insulin-Dependent Diabetes Mellitus, IDDM)

Type 1 diabetes mellitus results from **autoimmune destruction of pancreatic β-cells**, leading to **absolute insulin deficiency**. It usually occurs in **children and young adults**, though it may appear at any age. Genetic predisposition and environmental triggers such as viral infections play an important role. Patients are completely dependent on **exogenous insulin** for survival.

2. Type 2 Diabetes Mellitus (Non-Insulin-Dependent Diabetes Mellitus, NIDDM)

Type 2 diabetes mellitus is characterized by **insulin resistance** in peripheral tissues along with a **relative deficiency of insulin secretion**. It is the most common form of diabetes and typically occurs in **middle-aged and elderly individuals**, though its incidence is increasing in younger populations due to obesity and sedentary lifestyle. Both genetic and environmental factors contribute to its development.

3. Gestational Diabetes Mellitus (GDM)

Gestational diabetes mellitus is defined as **glucose intolerance first recognized during pregnancy**. It occurs due to increased insulin resistance caused by placental hormones. Although blood glucose levels usually return to normal after delivery, affected women have a higher risk of developing **Type 2 diabetes mellitus later in life**.

4. Other Specific Types of Diabetes

These include diabetes due to **genetic defects of β-cell function**, diseases of the pancreas, endocrinopathies, drug- or chemical-induced diabetes, and infections.

Etiology and Risk Factors

Type 1 Diabetes Mellitus

- Autoimmune destruction of β-cells
- Genetic susceptibility (HLA association)
- Environmental triggers such as viral infections

Type 2 Diabetes Mellitus

- Obesity and physical inactivity
- Genetic predisposition
- Aging
- Insulin resistance

- Unhealthy dietary habits

Pathophysiology of Diabetes Mellitus

Insulin Deficiency or Resistance: In diabetes mellitus, reduced insulin secretion or impaired insulin action leads to **decreased glucose uptake by muscle and adipose tissue**, while hepatic glucose production increases due to enhanced **gluconeogenesis and glycogenolysis**.

Hyperglycemia: Persistent elevation of blood glucose occurs due to:

- Reduced peripheral utilization of glucose
- Increased hepatic glucose output
- Reduced glycogen synthesis

Altered Fat Metabolism: Increased lipolysis results in elevated free fatty acids, which are converted into **ketone bodies** in the liver, especially in Type 1 diabetes. Excessive ketone production can lead to **diabetic ketoacidosis**.

Altered Protein Metabolism: Increased protein breakdown provides amino acids for gluconeogenesis, resulting in **muscle wasting and weight loss**.

Clinical Features of Diabetes Mellitus

Classical Symptoms

- Polyuria (excessive urination)
- Polydipsia (excessive thirst)
- Polyphagia (increased appetite)
- Weight loss (more prominent in Type 1 diabetes)

Other Symptoms

- Fatigue and weakness
- Blurred vision
- Recurrent infections
- Poor wound healing

Biochemical and Laboratory Findings

- Fasting plasma glucose ≥ 126 mg/dL
- Postprandial plasma glucose ≥ 200 mg/dL

- Random plasma glucose ≥ 200 mg/dL with symptoms
- HbA1c ≥ 6.5%
- Glycosuria and ketonuria in uncontrolled diabetes

Acute Complications of Diabetes Mellitus

Diabetic Ketoacidosis (DKA): Seen mainly in Type 1 diabetes, characterized by severe hyperglycemia, ketosis, metabolic acidosis, dehydration, and electrolyte imbalance.

Hyperosmolar Hyperglycemic State (HHS): Occurs primarily in Type 2 diabetes, marked by extreme hyperglycemia, severe dehydration, and absence of significant ketosis.

Hypoglycemia: May occur due to excess insulin or oral hypoglycemic drugs, presenting with sweating, tremors, confusion, and loss of consciousness.

Chronic Complications of Diabetes Mellitus

Microvascular Complications

- Diabetic retinopathy
- Diabetic nephropathy
- Diabetic neuropathy

Macrovascular Complications

- Coronary artery disease
- Cerebrovascular disease
- Peripheral vascular disease

Management of Diabetes Mellitus

Dietary Management

- Controlled carbohydrate intake
- High fiber diet
- Restriction of refined sugars and saturated fats

Physical Activity

- Improves insulin sensitivity
- Helps in weight management

Pharmacological Therapy

- Insulin therapy for Type 1 diabetes

- Oral hypoglycemic agents and injectable therapies for Type 2 diabetes

Monitoring

- Regular blood glucose monitoring
- Periodic HbA1c assessment

Chapter-4

Biological Oxidation

Biological oxidation is a fundamental biochemical process through which living cells obtain energy required for carrying out various physiological and metabolic activities essential for survival. In living systems, energy is not released by direct combustion of nutrients as occurs in non-living systems; instead, it is liberated in a controlled and stepwise manner through a series of enzyme-catalyzed oxidation–reduction reactions. These reactions collectively constitute biological oxidation and ensure efficient conservation of energy in a usable form, mainly as adenosine triphosphate (ATP).

In biological oxidation, electrons are removed from substrates such as carbohydrates, fats, and proteins and are ultimately transferred to molecular oxygen, which acts as the final electron acceptor. During this transfer, energy is released gradually and is utilized to synthesize ATP through processes such as oxidative phosphorylation. This controlled release of energy prevents cellular damage and allows cells to regulate their energy economy according to metabolic demands.

The major site of biological oxidation in eukaryotic cells is the mitochondrion, often referred to as the "powerhouse of the cell." Within mitochondria, a series of electron carriers organized into the electron transport chain facilitate the transfer of electrons from reduced coenzymes like NADH and $FADH_2$ to oxygen. The energy released during electron transfer is coupled with the formation of a proton gradient across the inner mitochondrial membrane, which drives ATP synthesis.

Biological oxidation plays a central role in metabolism by linking catabolic pathways such as glycolysis, citric acid cycle, and fatty acid oxidation with ATP generation. It also contributes to the maintenance of redox balance, regulation of metabolic pathways, and production of metabolic water. Any impairment in biological oxidation can lead to reduced energy production and is associated with several pathological conditions.

Thus, biological oxidation represents an essential and highly regulated process that enables living organisms to efficiently convert the chemical energy stored in nutrients into biologically useful energy, ensuring normal growth, development, and maintenance of cellular functions.

Electron Transport Chain (ETC)

The electron transport chain is an organized system of electron carriers that functions as the final pathway of biological oxidation and is responsible for the majority of ATP production in aerobic organisms. It operates by transferring electrons derived from metabolic fuels such as carbohydrates, fats, and proteins to molecular oxygen in a controlled and sequential manner. The electron transport chain is located on the inner mitochondrial membrane, whose structural integrity and selective permeability are essential for its proper functioning. The inner membrane forms folds called cristae, which increase the surface area available for the components of the electron transport chain and thereby enhance ATP synthesis.

The reduced coenzymes nicotinamide adenine dinucleotide (NADH) and flavin adenine dinucleotide ($FADH_2$), formed during glycolysis, oxidative decarboxylation of pyruvate, citric acid cycle, and β-oxidation of fatty acids, serve as the primary electron donors to the electron transport chain. These coenzymes carry high-energy electrons and transfer them to the electron carriers embedded in the inner mitochondrial membrane. The flow of electrons through the chain occurs in the direction of increasing redox potential, ensuring spontaneous and energy-yielding reactions.

Structural Organization of the Electron Transport Chain: The electron transport chain consists of four large multi-enzyme complexes, designated as Complex I to Complex IV, and two mobile electron carriers, namely coenzyme Q and cytochrome c. Each complex contains specific prosthetic groups such as flavins, iron–sulfur proteins, heme groups, and copper ions that participate in oxidation–reduction reactions. The complexes are arranged in a definite sequence that allows efficient transfer of electrons without loss of energy.

Complex I: NADH–Coenzyme Q Oxidoreductase: Complex I is the first and largest enzyme complex of the electron transport chain and serves as the entry point for electrons from NADH. It is composed of multiple subunits and contains flavin mononucleotide (FMN) as the initial electron acceptor along with several iron–sulfur (Fe–S) clusters. NADH transfers two electrons to FMN, forming $FMNH_2$. These electrons are then passed sequentially through the iron–sulfur centers and finally transferred to coenzyme Q. The oxidation of NADH to NAD^+ at this stage is essential for the continuation of metabolic pathways such as glycolysis and the citric acid cycle.

During electron transfer through Complex I, a significant amount of energy is released, which is utilized to pump protons from the mitochondrial matrix into the intermembrane space. This proton pumping contributes directly to the formation of the proton gradient that is required for ATP synthesis. Complex I is therefore one of the major sites of energy conservation in the electron transport chain.

Complex II: Succinate–Coenzyme Q Oxidoreductase: Complex II acts as a direct link between the citric acid cycle and the electron transport chain. It catalyzes the oxidation of succinate to fumarate in the citric acid cycle and contains flavin adenine dinucleotide (FAD) as a tightly bound prosthetic group. During this reaction, FAD is reduced to $FADH_2$, which subsequently donates its electrons to iron–sulfur proteins within the complex and finally to coenzyme Q.

Unlike Complex I, Complex II does not pump protons across the inner mitochondrial membrane. As a result, electrons entering the electron transport chain through Complex II generate less ATP compared to electrons entering through Complex I. This difference explains the lower

ATP yield from $FADH_2$ compared to NADH.

Coenzyme Q (Ubiquinone): Coenzyme Q is a lipid-soluble, non-protein electron carrier that is freely mobile within the hydrophobic core of the inner mitochondrial membrane. It plays a central role in the electron transport chain by accepting electrons from Complex I, Complex II, and other flavoprotein dehydrogenases such as those involved in fatty acid oxidation. Coenzyme Q can exist in three oxidation states: oxidized ubiquinone, partially reduced semiquinone, and fully reduced ubiquinol. This ability allows it to effectively transfer electrons between complexes with different electron-carrying capacities.

Complex III: Coenzyme Q–Cytochrome c Oxidoreductase: Complex III transfers electrons from reduced coenzyme Q to cytochrome c and contains cytochromes b and c_1 as well as iron–sulfur proteins. Electron transfer within Complex III occurs through a specialized mechanism known as the Q cycle, which allows efficient transfer of electrons while simultaneously pumping protons across the inner mitochondrial membrane. During this process, electrons are split and transferred in a stepwise fashion, leading to the movement of protons from the matrix to the intermembrane space.

The Q cycle is an important amplification mechanism because it enables the release of additional protons, thereby strengthening the proton gradient and enhancing ATP synthesis.

Cytochrome c: Cytochrome c is a small, water-soluble heme protein that is loosely associated with the outer surface of the inner mitochondrial membrane. It functions as a mobile electron carrier that transfers one electron at a time from Complex III to Complex IV. The presence of iron in its heme group allows cytochrome c to alternate between reduced and oxidized states, ensuring continuous electron flow. Cytochrome c also plays a role in apoptosis when released into the cytosol, highlighting its significance beyond energy metabolism.

Complex IV: Cytochrome c Oxidase: Complex IV is the terminal complex of the electron transport chain and is responsible for the transfer of electrons from cytochrome c to molecular oxygen. It contains cytochromes a and a_3 along with copper ions that facilitate electron transfer. Oxygen acts as the final electron acceptor and is reduced to water by accepting electrons and protons. This reaction is essential for maintaining the flow of electrons through the chain and for preventing the accumulation of reduced electron carriers.

Complex IV also contributes to proton pumping across the inner mitochondrial membrane, further reinforcing the proton motive force. The reduction of oxygen to water marks the completion of the electron transport process.

Mechanism of Electron Transport Chain

The mechanism of the electron transport chain involves a continuous flow of electrons from reduced coenzymes to oxygen through a series of redox reactions. Electrons from NADH enter the chain at Complex I, while electrons from $FADH_2$ enter at Complex II. These electrons are transferred sequentially through coenzyme Q, Complex III, cytochrome c, and Complex IV, finally reducing oxygen to water.

As electrons move through the chain, energy is released at specific points, namely at Complex I, Complex III, and Complex IV. This energy is used to pump protons from the mitochondrial matrix into the intermembrane space, creating an electrochemical gradient composed of both a proton concentration gradient and a membrane potential. This gradient stores potential energy in the form of the proton motive force.

The proton motive force drives protons back into the mitochondrial matrix through ATP synthase, a large enzyme complex located in the inner mitochondrial membrane. The movement of protons through ATP synthase induces conformational changes that catalyze the synthesis of ATP from ADP and inorganic phosphate. This coupling of electron transfer with ATP formation is known as oxidative phosphorylation.

Oxidative Phosphorylation

Oxidative phosphorylation is the biochemical process by which energy released during the oxidation of reduced coenzymes in the electron transport chain is utilized for the synthesis of adenosine triphosphate. It represents the final stage of cellular respiration and is the major source of ATP in aerobic organisms. In this process, oxidation of NADH and $FADH_2$ is tightly coupled with phosphorylation of adenosine diphosphate to ATP, hence the term oxidative phosphorylation. The process occurs on the inner mitochondrial membrane, whose unique structure and impermeability to ions are essential for effective energy conservation.

Oxidative phosphorylation links electron transport with ATP synthesis through the generation of an electrochemical proton gradient. As electrons flow through the electron transport chain, protons are pumped from the mitochondrial matrix into the intermembrane space, creating a difference in proton concentration and electrical charge across the inner membrane. This gradient stores energy that is later used to drive ATP synthesis.

Components Involved in Oxidative Phosphorylation: Oxidative phosphorylation requires the coordinated functioning of the electron transport chain, the inner mitochondrial membrane, molecular oxygen, and ATP synthase. The inner mitochondrial membrane acts as a barrier that prevents free diffusion of protons, allowing the establishment of a proton gradient. ATP synthase, also known as Complex V, is the enzyme responsible for ATP formation. It consists of two major functional units, F_0 and F_1, which work together to convert the energy of the proton gradient into chemical energy stored in ATP.

ATP Synthase (Complex V): ATP synthase is a large multisubunit enzyme complex embedded in the inner mitochondrial membrane. The F_0 portion is membrane-bound and forms a proton channel, while the F_1 portion projects into the mitochondrial matrix and contains the catalytic sites for ATP synthesis. The F_0 unit allows protons to flow back into the matrix, and this proton movement induces rotational and conformational changes in the F_1 unit. These changes enable the binding of ADP and inorganic phosphate, their condensation to form ATP, and the release of newly synthesized ATP.

Mechanism of Oxidative Phosphorylation

The mechanism of oxidative phosphorylation is best explained by the chemiosmotic theory proposed by Peter Mitchell. According to this theory, the transfer of electrons through the electron transport chain leads to the pumping of protons across the inner mitochondrial membrane at specific sites. This proton pumping generates a proton motive force consisting of a pH gradient and an electrical potential difference across the membrane.

As protons accumulate in the intermembrane space, they create a state of high potential energy. The inner mitochondrial membrane is impermeable to protons, so they can return to the matrix only through the F_0 channel of ATP synthase. The movement of protons through this channel causes rotation of the F_0 subunit and the central stalk of the enzyme, which in turn induces conformational changes in the β subunits of the F_1 portion.

The F_1 portion of ATP synthase operates through a binding change mechanism, in which the β subunits alternate between three conformations: loose, tight, and open. In the loose conformation, ADP and inorganic phosphate bind to the enzyme. In the tight conformation, ATP is synthesized from ADP and phosphate. In the open conformation, the newly formed ATP is released into the mitochondrial matrix. Each complete rotation of the enzyme results in the synthesis of multiple ATP molecules.

Role of Oxygen in Oxidative Phosphorylation: Oxygen plays a critical role in oxidative phosphorylation by acting as the final electron acceptor in the electron transport chain. At Complex IV, oxygen accepts electrons and combines with protons to form water. This reaction maintains the flow of electrons through the chain and prevents the accumulation of reduced electron carriers. In the absence of oxygen, electron transport and oxidative phosphorylation come to a halt, leading to cessation of ATP production and eventual cell death.

Energy Yield of Oxidative Phosphorylation: The energy yield of oxidative phosphorylation depends on the number of protons pumped across the membrane and the efficiency of ATP synthase. Oxidation of one molecule of NADH generally leads to the synthesis of approximately three ATP molecules, while oxidation of one molecule of $FADH_2$ yields about two ATP molecules. This difference is due to the entry of electrons at different points in the electron transport chain.

Significance of Oxidative Phosphorylation: Oxidative phosphorylation is of immense biological importance as it provides the energy required for various cellular processes such as biosynthesis, active transport, muscle contraction, nerve impulse transmission, and maintenance of cellular integrity. It also plays a role in thermoregulation and metabolic regulation. Any defect in oxidative phosphorylation can lead to decreased ATP production and is associated with several metabolic and mitochondrial disorders.

Substrate Level Phosphorylation

Substrate level phosphorylation is a metabolic process in which adenosine triphosphate is synthesized directly by the transfer of a high-energy phosphate group from a phosphorylated substrate to adenosine diphosphate. In this process, ATP formation occurs independently of the electron transport chain and oxidative phosphorylation. It represents one of the simplest and most direct mechanisms of ATP generation in living cells and plays a crucial role, especially under conditions where oxygen supply is limited or mitochondrial function is impaired.

Unlike oxidative phosphorylation, substrate level phosphorylation does not require molecular oxygen, an intact mitochondrial membrane, or a proton gradient. The energy required for ATP synthesis is derived directly from the cleavage of a high-energy phosphate bond present in a metabolic intermediate. This process occurs in the cytosol as well as in the mitochondrial matrix, depending on the metabolic pathway involved.

Mechanism of Substrate Level Phosphorylation

The mechanism of substrate level phosphorylation involves the formation of a high-energy phosphorylated intermediate during a metabolic reaction. This intermediate possesses sufficient free energy to donate its phosphate group directly to ADP, resulting in the formation of ATP. The reaction is catalyzed by specific enzymes known as kinases, which facilitate the transfer of the phosphate group.

In this mechanism, the phosphorylated substrate binds to the active site of the enzyme along with ADP. The enzyme then catalyzes the transfer of the phosphate group from the substrate to ADP, producing ATP and a dephosphorylated product. The energy released during the conversion of the high-energy substrate to a lower-energy product drives ATP synthesis.

Sites of Substrate Level Phosphorylation: Substrate level phosphorylation occurs at specific steps in major metabolic pathways. In glycolysis, ATP is generated during the conversion of 1,3-bisphosphoglycerate to 3-phosphoglycerate, catalyzed by phosphoglycerate kinase, and during the conversion of phosphoenolpyruvate to pyruvate, catalyzed by pyruvate kinase. These reactions take place in the cytosol and provide a rapid source of ATP.

In the citric acid cycle, substrate level phosphorylation occurs during the conversion of succinyl-CoA to succinate, catalyzed by succinyl-CoA synthetase. In this reaction, guanosine diphosphate is phosphorylated to guanosine triphosphate, which can subsequently transfer its phosphate group to ADP to form ATP. This reaction takes place in the mitochondrial matrix.

Energy Yield of Substrate Level Phosphorylation: The amount of ATP generated by substrate level phosphorylation is relatively small compared to oxidative phosphorylation. During glycolysis, a net gain of two ATP molecules is achieved per molecule of glucose through substrate level phosphorylation. In the citric acid cycle, one molecule of GTP, equivalent to one ATP, is produced per turn of the cycle. Despite its lower yield, substrate level phosphorylation is vital because it provides ATP rapidly and does not depend on oxygen availability.

Significance of Substrate Level Phosphorylation: Substrate level phosphorylation is particularly important under anaerobic conditions or in tissues with limited mitochondrial activity, such as red blood cells, which lack mitochondria entirely. In such cells, substrate level phosphorylation is the only source of ATP. It also plays a key role during intense muscular activity when oxygen supply may be insufficient to meet energy demands through oxidative phosphorylation alone.

Inhibitors of Electron Transport Chain (ETC)

Inhibitors of the electron transport chain are substances that interfere with the normal flow of electrons through the respiratory chain. These inhibitors block electron transfer at specific sites within the chain, thereby preventing oxidation of reduced coenzymes and impairing ATP synthesis. Since the electron transport chain is the major source of energy in aerobic cells, inhibition of this process leads to decreased ATP production and can result in cellular dysfunction or death. The study of ETC inhibitors is important in understanding the mechanism of biological oxidation as well as the toxic effects of certain drugs and poisons.

Inhibitors of Complex I (NADH–Coenzyme Q Oxidoreductase): Complex I inhibitors block the transfer of electrons from NADH to coenzyme Q. As a result, oxidation of NADH is prevented, leading to accumulation of NADH and reduced regeneration of NAD^+. This affects metabolic pathways such as glycolysis and the citric acid cycle, which depend on NAD^+ for their continuation. Rotenone, a plant-derived insecticide, is a classic inhibitor of Complex I. It binds to the iron–sulfur proteins of the complex and prevents electron transfer to coenzyme Q. Amobarbital, a barbiturate, also inhibits electron flow at Complex I by interfering with the transfer of electrons from FMN to coenzyme Q. Piericidin A, an antibiotic, acts in a similar manner by blocking the NADH dehydrogenase component of the complex.

Inhibitors of Complex II (Succinate–Coenzyme Q Oxidoreductase): Complex II inhibitors prevent the transfer of electrons from succinate to coenzyme Q. Malonate is a well-known competitive inhibitor of succinate dehydrogenase and structurally resembles succinate. By competing with succinate for the active site of the enzyme, malonate inhibits the oxidation of succinate to fumarate and consequently reduces electron entry into the electron transport chain through $FADH_2$. Although inhibition of Complex II reduces ATP production, its effect is less severe compared to inhibition of Complex I because electrons from NADH can still enter the chain.

Inhibitors of Complex III (Coenzyme Q–Cytochrome c Oxidoreductase): Complex III inhibitors block electron transfer from reduced coenzyme Q to cytochrome c. Antimycin A is a potent inhibitor of Complex III that binds to the cytochrome b component of the complex and prevents electron flow through the Q cycle. This leads to accumulation of reduced coenzyme Q and cessation of proton pumping at this site, thereby decreasing the proton gradient and ATP synthesis.

Inhibitors of Complex IV (Cytochrome c Oxidase): Complex IV inhibitors are among the most lethal ETC inhibitors because they block the final step of electron transfer to molecular oxygen. Cyanide is a highly toxic compound that binds to the ferric form of iron in cytochrome a_3, preventing the reduction of oxygen to water. Carbon monoxide also inhibits Complex IV by binding to the ferrous form of iron in cytochrome a_3, thereby blocking oxygen binding. Sodium azide acts in a similar manner by inhibiting cytochrome c oxidase. Inhibition of Complex IV causes complete cessation of electron transport and oxidative phosphorylation, leading to rapid depletion of ATP and cellular hypoxia despite adequate oxygen availability.

Inhibitors of ATP Synthase (Complex V): Some inhibitors directly affect ATP synthase and prevent ATP formation without directly inhibiting electron transport. Oligomycin is a classic inhibitor of ATP synthase that binds to the F_0 portion and blocks the proton channel. This prevents the flow of protons back into the mitochondrial matrix, thereby inhibiting ATP synthesis. As proton accumulation increases in the intermembrane space, electron transport also slows down due to increased resistance to proton pumping.

Physiological and Clinical Significance of ETC Inhibitors: Inhibitors of the electron transport chain are valuable tools in biochemical research for studying mitochondrial function and energy metabolism. Clinically, exposure to ETC inhibitors such as cyanide and carbon monoxide leads to severe energy deficiency and can be fatal if not treated promptly. Some inhibitors have therapeutic applications at controlled doses, while others are used as pesticides or research agents. Understanding the sites and mechanisms of ETC inhibition is essential for recognizing their metabolic consequences and toxicological effects.

Uncouplers of Oxidative Phosphorylation

Uncouplers of oxidative phosphorylation are substances that disrupt the normal coupling between electron transport and ATP synthesis. In the presence of uncouplers, electron transport through the respiratory chain continues normally, and oxygen consumption may even increase, but the energy released during electron transfer is not utilized for ATP synthesis. Instead, this energy is dissipated as heat. Thus, uncouplers separate or "uncouple" oxidative processes from phosphorylation, leading to reduced or absent ATP formation despite active electron transport.

Under normal conditions, the proton gradient generated by the electron transport chain drives protons back into the mitochondrial matrix through ATP synthase, resulting in ATP synthesis. Uncouplers interfere with this process by increasing the permeability of the inner mitochondrial membrane to protons or by bypassing ATP synthase, thereby collapsing the proton gradient. As a result, the proton motive force is dissipated, and ATP synthesis is inhibited.

Mechanism of Action of Uncouplers: The primary mechanism of uncouplers involves the dissipation of the proton gradient across the inner mitochondrial membrane. Most chemical uncouplers are lipid-soluble weak acids that can shuttle protons across the membrane. In their protonated form, they diffuse through the inner mitochondrial membrane from the intermembrane space into the matrix. Once inside the matrix, they release the proton and return to the intermembrane space in their unprotonated form to repeat the cycle. This continuous proton leakage prevents the buildup of a proton gradient required for ATP synthesis.

Because the proton gradient is reduced or eliminated, ATP synthase is unable to function effectively. However, electron transport continues, and in an attempt to re-establish the proton gradient, the respiratory chain operates at an increased rate. This leads to increased oxidation of NADH and $FADH_2$ and increased oxygen consumption, but ATP production remains low. The excess energy released during electron transfer is converted into heat.

Chemical Uncouplers of Oxidative Phosphorylation: Several chemical agents act as uncouplers of oxidative phosphorylation. 2,4-dinitrophenol is a classical uncoupler that increases the permeability of the inner mitochondrial membrane to protons. It was once used as a weight-reducing agent due to its ability to increase metabolic rate and heat production, but its use was discontinued because of severe toxicity. Other chemical uncouplers include carbonyl cyanide p-trifluoromethoxyphenylhydrazone and carbonyl cyanide m-chlorophenylhydrazone, which are potent protonophores used mainly in research.

Certain drugs and toxins, such as high doses of salicylates, also exhibit uncoupling effects by disrupting the proton gradient. These agents cause increased heat production and can lead to hyperthermia if present in excessive amounts.

Physiological Uncouplers: Uncoupling of oxidative phosphorylation also occurs under physiological conditions. Thermogenin, also known as uncoupling protein 1, is present in the inner mitochondrial membrane of brown adipose tissue. It provides a pathway for protons to re-enter the mitochondrial matrix without passing through ATP synthase. The energy of the proton gradient is thus released as heat, which is important for thermoregulation, especially in newborns and hibernating animals.

Other uncoupling proteins present in various tissues may play roles in regulating metabolic efficiency, reducing reactive oxygen species formation, and adapting energy metabolism to physiological needs.

Effects of Uncouplers on Cellular Metabolism: The presence of uncouplers leads to decreased ATP levels, increased oxygen consumption, and enhanced oxidation of metabolic fuels. Cells respond by increasing the rate of substrate oxidation in an attempt to maintain ATP levels. Prolonged or severe uncoupling can result in energy depletion, impaired cellular function, and cell death. Increased heat production is a characteristic feature of uncoupling and can be beneficial in thermogenesis but harmful in cases of poisoning.

Difference Between Uncouplers and ETC Inhibitors: Uncouplers differ from electron transport chain inhibitors in that they do not block electron flow. In fact, electron transport continues or accelerates in the presence of uncouplers. In contrast, ETC inhibitors prevent electron transfer at specific sites, leading to decreased oxygen consumption and ATP synthesis. Thus, while both uncouplers and inhibitors reduce ATP production, their mechanisms and metabolic consequences are distinct.

Chapter-5

Lipid Metabolism

Lipid metabolism refers to the complex set of biochemical processes involved in the digestion, absorption, transport, synthesis, degradation and utilization of lipids in the human body. Lipids are a major class of biomolecules that include fats, oils, phospholipids, glycolipids, sterols and fat-soluble vitamins. They serve as a concentrated source of energy, structural components of cell membranes, precursors of biologically active molecules and essential regulators of various physiological functions. Because lipids are hydrophobic in nature, their metabolism involves specialized mechanisms and transport systems distinct from those of carbohydrates and proteins.

From a biochemical point of view, lipid metabolism encompasses two broad aspects, namely lipid catabolism and lipid anabolism. Lipid catabolism mainly involves the breakdown of dietary and stored lipids to release energy, particularly through processes such as lipolysis and β-oxidation of fatty acids. Lipid anabolism includes the synthesis of fatty acids, triglycerides, phospholipids, cholesterol and other complex lipids required for normal cellular structure and function. These anabolic and catabolic pathways are highly regulated and interconnected with carbohydrate and protein metabolism, ensuring metabolic balance in the body.

Dietary lipids are primarily consumed in the form of triglycerides, along with smaller amounts of phospholipids and cholesterol. During digestion, these lipids are emulsified, hydrolyzed and absorbed in the intestine, after which they are transported through the bloodstream in the form of lipoproteins. Once delivered to tissues, lipids may be stored in adipose tissue as triglycerides, oxidized to meet energy demands, or utilized for the synthesis of cellular membranes, hormones and signaling molecules. The liver plays a central role in lipid metabolism by coordinating lipid synthesis, modification, distribution and degradation.

Lipid metabolism is of great physiological and clinical importance. Fatty acids provide more than twice the energy per gram compared to carbohydrates and proteins, making lipids the most efficient energy reserves of the body. In addition, lipids are essential for the absorption of fat-soluble vitamins (A, D, E and K), maintenance of membrane integrity, insulation of nerve fibers and protection of vital organs. Disturbances in lipid metabolism can lead to various metabolic disorders such as obesity, hyperlipidemia, atherosclerosis, fatty liver disease and cardiovascular complications, which highlights the importance of understanding lipid metabolic pathways.

β-Oxidation of Saturated Fatty Acid (Palmitic Acid)

β-Oxidation is the principal pathway for the degradation of saturated fatty acids in the body, through which fatty acids are oxidized in a stepwise manner to produce energy. This process occurs mainly in the mitochondrial matrix of cells, particularly in tissues with high energy demands such as liver, heart, skeletal muscle and kidney. Palmitic acid, a saturated fatty acid containing 16 carbon atoms, is commonly used as the classical example to explain the mechanism and energetics of β-oxidation.

Definition and Significance of β-Oxidation: β-Oxidation is a cyclic metabolic process in which fatty acids are broken down by the successive removal of two-carbon units in the form of acetyl-CoA. The name β-oxidation is derived from the fact that oxidation occurs at the β-carbon (the third carbon atom from the carboxyl end) of the fatty acid chain. The acetyl-CoA produced enters the citric acid cycle for further oxidation, leading to the generation of large amounts of ATP. Thus, β-oxidation plays a crucial role in energy production, especially during fasting, prolonged exercise and low-carbohydrate states.

Activation of Palmitic Acid: Before palmitic acid can undergo β-oxidation, it must be activated in the cytosol. This activation involves the conversion of free palmitic acid into palmitoyl-CoA. The reaction is catalyzed by the enzyme fatty acyl-CoA synthetase (also called thiokinase) and requires ATP and coenzyme A. In this process, ATP is converted to AMP and inorganic pyrophosphate, which is equivalent to the utilization of two high-energy phosphate bonds. Activation is an essential step because only fatty acyl-CoA can enter the β-oxidation pathway.

Transport of Palmitoyl-CoA into Mitochondria (Carnitine Shuttle): Long-chain fatty acids such as palmitic acid cannot cross the inner mitochondrial membrane directly. Therefore, a specialized transport system known as the carnitine shuttle is required. In the outer mitochondrial membrane, palmitoyl-CoA combines with carnitine in a reaction catalyzed by carnitine acyltransferase I (CAT-I), forming palmitoyl-carnitine. This molecule is transported across the inner mitochondrial membrane by a translocase. Inside the mitochondrial matrix, palmitoyl-carnitine is converted back to palmitoyl-CoA by carnitine acyltransferase II (CAT-II), releasing free carnitine, which returns to the cytosol. This transport step is highly regulated and represents an important control point in fatty acid oxidation.

Steps of β-Oxidation of Palmitic Acid: Once inside the mitochondrial matrix, palmitoyl-CoA undergoes a series of four recurring reactions that constitute one cycle of β-oxidation. Each cycle shortens the fatty acid chain by two carbon atoms and generates energy-rich molecules.

The first step is oxidation. Palmitoyl-CoA is oxidized by the enzyme acyl-CoA dehydrogenase, forming trans-Δ^2-enoyl-CoA. In this reaction, FAD is reduced to $FADH_2$, which later donates electrons to the electron transport chain for ATP synthesis.

The second step is hydration. Trans-Δ^2-enoyl-CoA undergoes hydration in the presence of the enzyme enoyl-CoA hydratase, resulting in the formation of L-β-hydroxyacyl-CoA.

The third step is a second oxidation. L-β-hydroxyacyl-CoA is oxidized by β-hydroxyacyl-CoA dehydrogenase to form β-ketoacyl-CoA. In this reaction, NAD^+ is reduced to NADH, which also contributes to ATP production via the electron transport chain.

The fourth and final step is thiolysis. β-Ketoacyl-CoA undergoes cleavage by the enzyme thiolase in the presence of coenzyme A, releasing one molecule of acetyl-CoA and a fatty acyl-CoA shortened by two carbon atoms. The shortened fatty acyl-CoA then re-enters the β-oxidation cycle.

β-Oxidation Cycles and Products of Palmitic Acid: Palmitic acid contains 16 carbon atoms. During β-oxidation, it undergoes seven cycles of oxidation. Each cycle removes two carbon atoms as acetyl-CoA. As a result, complete β-oxidation of palmitic acid yields eight molecules of acetyl-CoA, seven molecules of $FADH_2$ and seven molecules of NADH. The acetyl-CoA molecules enter the citric acid cycle, while NADH and $FADH_2$ are oxidized in the electron transport chain to generate ATP.

Energetics of β-Oxidation of Palmitic Acid: The energy yield from the complete oxidation of palmitic acid is very high. Each $FADH_2$ produces approximately 2 ATP and each NADH produces approximately 3 ATP through oxidative phosphorylation. Therefore, seven $FADH_2$ yield about 14 ATP and seven NADH yield about 21 ATP. The eight acetyl-CoA molecules produced enter the citric acid cycle, where each acetyl-CoA generates about 12 ATP, resulting in a total of 96 ATP. Thus, the gross ATP yield from palmitic acid oxidation is 131 ATP. Since two ATP equivalents are consumed during the activation of palmitic acid, the net ATP yield is approximately 129 ATP.

Regulation of β-Oxidation: β-Oxidation is tightly regulated to meet the energy requirements of the body. The most important regulatory step is the transport of fatty acids into the mitochondria via carnitine acyltransferase I. This enzyme is inhibited by malonyl-CoA, an intermediate of fatty acid synthesis, thereby preventing simultaneous synthesis and degradation of fatty acids. Hormonal regulation also plays a role, with glucagon and adrenaline promoting fatty acid oxidation, while insulin inhibits it by favoring lipid synthesis.

Physiological and Clinical Importance: β-Oxidation of fatty acids, particularly palmitic acid, is a major source of energy during fasting, starvation and prolonged physical activity. Efficient β-oxidation helps maintain blood glucose levels by sparing glucose for tissues that depend on it, such as the brain and red blood cells. Defects in enzymes involved in β-oxidation or in the carnitine transport system can lead to serious metabolic disorders characterized by hypoglycemia, muscle weakness and accumulation of fatty acids. Therefore, understanding the β-oxidation of saturated fatty acids is essential for appreciating normal energy metabolism as well as the biochemical basis of related diseases and their pharmacological management.

Formation and Utilization of Ketone Bodies; Ketoacidosis

Ketone bodies are water-soluble compounds produced in the liver from fatty acids during conditions in which carbohydrate availability is limited and fatty acid oxidation is increased. The process of formation of ketone bodies is known as ketogenesis, while their utilization by peripheral tissues is called ketolysis. Ketone bodies serve as an important alternative source of energy, particularly for extrahepatic tissues such as brain, heart and skeletal muscles during prolonged fasting and starvation. However, excessive production and accumulation of ketone bodies in blood can lead to a serious metabolic condition known as ketoacidosis.

Ketone Bodies and Their Types: Ketone bodies are three chemically related compounds formed in the liver mitochondria. These include acetoacetic acid, β-hydroxybutyric acid and acetone. Acetoacetic acid is the primary ketone body synthesized, β-hydroxybutyric acid is formed by the reduction of acetoacetic acid and acetone is produced by spontaneous decarboxylation of acetoacetic acid. Among these, acetoacetate and β-hydroxybutyrate are physiologically important and serve as major energy sources, while acetone is largely excreted through the lungs, giving a characteristic fruity odor to the breath.

Formation of Ketone Bodies (Ketogenesis): Ketogenesis occurs exclusively in the mitochondrial matrix of liver cells. Under normal conditions, acetyl-CoA formed from β-oxidation of fatty acids enters the citric acid cycle. However, during fasting, starvation, uncontrolled diabetes mellitus or low-carbohydrate intake, the availability of oxaloacetate is reduced because it is diverted toward gluconeogenesis. As a result, acetyl-CoA accumulates in the liver mitochondria and is channeled into the pathway of ketone body formation.

The first step in ketogenesis involves the condensation of two molecules of acetyl-CoA to form acetoacetyl-CoA, catalyzed by the enzyme thiolase. In the next step, acetoacetyl-CoA condenses with another molecule of acetyl-CoA to form β-hydroxy-β-methylglutaryl-CoA (HMG-CoA). This reaction is catalyzed by HMG-CoA synthase, which is the rate-limiting and key regulatory enzyme of ketone body formation. HMG-CoA is then cleaved by HMG-CoA lyase to yield acetoacetic acid and acetyl-CoA. Acetoacetic acid can either be reduced to β-hydroxybutyric acid in the presence of NADH or undergo spontaneous decarboxylation to form acetone. The ketone bodies thus formed are released into the bloodstream and transported to peripheral tissues.

Utilization of Ketone Bodies (Ketolysis): Ketone bodies are utilized by extrahepatic tissues such as skeletal muscle, cardiac muscle, renal cortex and brain during prolonged fasting. The liver itself cannot utilize ketone bodies because it lacks the enzyme succinyl-CoA: acetoacetate CoA transferase (also known as thiophorase), which is essential for ketone body utilization.

In peripheral tissues, β-hydroxybutyric acid is first oxidized to acetoacetic acid by β-hydroxybutyrate dehydrogenase. Acetoacetic acid then reacts with succinyl-CoA in a reaction catalyzed by thiophorase, forming acetoacetyl-CoA. This step bypasses the need for ATP. Acetoacetyl-CoA is subsequently cleaved by thiolase to produce two molecules of acetyl-CoA. These acetyl-CoA molecules enter the citric acid cycle and are completely oxidized to carbon dioxide and water, producing ATP. Thus, ketone bodies act as efficient fuels for peripheral tissues during periods of increased fat metabolism.

Energetic Significance of Ketone Bodies: Ketone bodies are an important energy source during prolonged fasting and starvation. Oxidation of one molecule of acetoacetic acid yields approximately 24 ATP, while oxidation of one molecule of β-hydroxybutyric acid yields about 27 ATP due to the additional NADH generated during its conversion to acetoacetate. In prolonged fasting, the brain gradually adapts to utilize ketone bodies, thereby reducing its dependence on glucose and conserving body protein by decreasing the need for gluconeogenesis from amino acids.

Regulation of Ketone Body Formation: Ketogenesis is regulated primarily by the rate of fatty acid mobilization from adipose tissue and the availability of acetyl-CoA in the liver. Hormonal factors play a major role, with insulin inhibiting ketone body formation and glucagon, adrenaline and cortisol promoting it. Low insulin levels increase lipolysis in adipose tissue, leading to increased free fatty acid supply to the liver and enhanced β-oxidation. Increased $NADH/NAD^+$ ratio in the liver favors the formation of β-hydroxybutyric acid from acetoacetic acid.

Ketoacidosis: Ketoacidosis is a pathological condition characterized by excessive accumulation of ketone bodies in the blood, resulting in metabolic acidosis. It is most commonly seen in uncontrolled type 1 diabetes mellitus, prolonged starvation and chronic alcoholism. In diabetic ketoacidosis, absolute or relative insulin deficiency leads to increased lipolysis and excessive hepatic ketone body production. The buffering capacity of blood is overwhelmed by the acidic ketone bodies, leading to a decrease in blood pH.

Clinically, ketoacidosis is characterized by hyperglycemia, ketonemia, ketonuria, dehydration, electrolyte imbalance and metabolic acidosis. Patients may present with symptoms such as polyuria, polydipsia, nausea, vomiting, abdominal pain, deep and rapid breathing known as

Kussmaul respiration and a fruity odor of breath due to acetone. If untreated, ketoacidosis can progress to coma and death.

Biochemical and Clinical Importance: The formation and utilization of ketone bodies represent an important metabolic adaptation that allows survival during periods of carbohydrate deprivation. However, excessive ketone body production can have serious clinical consequences. Understanding the biochemical basis of ketogenesis, ketolysis and ketoacidosis is essential for pharmacy students, as it provides insight into the pathophysiology of diabetes mellitus and forms the basis for therapeutic strategies aimed at controlling blood glucose levels and preventing metabolic complications.

De novo Synthesis of Fatty Acids (Palmitic Acid)

De novo synthesis of fatty acids refers to the formation of fatty acids from non-lipid precursors, mainly carbohydrates, in the body. This process is of particular importance when dietary intake of fat is low and there is an excess of carbohydrate and energy. The major product of de novo fatty acid synthesis in humans is palmitic acid, a saturated fatty acid containing 16 carbon atoms. Fatty acid synthesis is an anabolic process that occurs primarily in the liver, adipose tissue, lactating mammary glands and, to a lesser extent, in kidneys and brain.

Site and Cellular Compartment of Fatty Acid Synthesis: Unlike β-oxidation, which takes place in the mitochondrial matrix, de novo fatty acid synthesis occurs in the cytosol of cells. However, the acetyl-CoA required for fatty acid synthesis is generated in the mitochondria during carbohydrate metabolism. Since acetyl-CoA cannot cross the mitochondrial membrane directly, it is transported to the cytosol in the form of citrate through the citrate shuttle mechanism. In the cytosol, citrate is cleaved by ATP-citrate lyase to regenerate acetyl-CoA and oxaloacetate, thus providing the substrate for fatty acid synthesis.

Source of Acetyl-CoA and NADPH: Acetyl-CoA serves as the basic building block for fatty acid synthesis. The acetyl-CoA used for this purpose is derived mainly from glucose metabolism via glycolysis and pyruvate oxidation. In addition to acetyl-CoA, fatty acid synthesis requires a large amount of reducing power in the form of NADPH. NADPH is supplied primarily by the pentose phosphate pathway and also by the malic enzyme, which converts malate to pyruvate in the cytosol while generating NADPH. Thus, carbohydrate metabolism and fatty acid synthesis are closely linked.

Formation of Malonyl-CoA: The first and committed step in fatty acid synthesis is the carboxylation of acetyl-CoA to form malonyl-CoA. This reaction is catalyzed by the enzyme acetyl-CoA carboxylase, which requires biotin as a coenzyme and ATP as a source of energy. Carbon dioxide provides the carboxyl group, which is temporarily added to acetyl-CoA. This step is highly regulated and represents the rate-limiting step of fatty acid synthesis. Malonyl-CoA serves as the two-carbon donor for chain elongation during fatty acid synthesis.

Fatty Acid Synthase Complex: The synthesis of palmitic acid is carried out by a multifunctional enzyme complex known as fatty acid synthase. This large cytosolic enzyme contains multiple enzymatic activities and an acyl carrier protein (ACP) domain that holds the growing fatty acid chain. ACP contains a phosphopantetheine group derived from vitamin pantothenic acid, which acts as a flexible arm to transfer intermediates between active sites of the enzyme complex.

Steps in the Synthesis of Palmitic Acid: Fatty acid synthesis proceeds through a repeating cycle of reactions, each cycle adding two carbon atoms to the growing fatty acid chain. The process begins with the attachment of an acetyl group from acetyl-CoA to the ACP, which serves as the primer. A malonyl group from malonyl-CoA is then transferred to ACP. The acetyl and malonyl groups undergo a condensation reaction, releasing carbon dioxide and forming a four-carbon β-ketoacyl-ACP.

The β-ketoacyl-ACP formed is subsequently reduced to β-hydroxyacyl-ACP by β-ketoacyl-ACP reductase using NADPH as a reducing agent. This is followed by dehydration by β-hydroxyacyl-ACP dehydratase to form an enoyl-ACP. The enoyl-ACP is then reduced by enoyl-ACP reductase, again using NADPH, to form a saturated acyl-ACP. This saturated acyl-ACP re-enters the cycle, where it condenses with another malonyl-ACP molecule, leading to chain elongation.

This cycle of condensation, reduction, dehydration and reduction is repeated until a 16-carbon saturated fatty acid chain is formed. After seven cycles of elongation, palmitoyl-ACP is produced, which is then hydrolyzed by the enzyme thioesterase to release free palmitic acid.

Overall Reaction and Stoichiometry: The overall synthesis of palmitic acid requires one molecule of acetyl-CoA as a primer and seven molecules of malonyl-CoA for chain elongation. Since each malonyl-CoA molecule is formed from acetyl-CoA, a total of eight molecules of acetyl-CoA are required. The process also consumes seven molecules of ATP during the formation of malonyl-CoA and fourteen molecules of NADPH during the reduction steps. Thus, fatty acid synthesis is an energy-intensive process that occurs when energy and substrate availability are high.

Regulation of Fatty Acid Synthesis: Fatty acid synthesis is tightly regulated to maintain metabolic balance. Acetyl-CoA carboxylase is the key regulatory enzyme and is activated by citrate, which signals an abundance of acetyl-CoA and energy. It is inhibited by long-chain fatty acyl-CoA, such as palmitoyl-CoA, through feedback inhibition. Hormonal regulation also plays a significant role, with insulin stimulating fatty acid synthesis by increasing the activity and expression of lipogenic enzymes, while glucagon and adrenaline inhibit fatty acid synthesis by decreasing acetyl-CoA carboxylase activity through phosphorylation.

Malonyl-CoA also plays a regulatory role by inhibiting carnitine acyltransferase I, thereby preventing simultaneous fatty acid synthesis and β-oxidation. This ensures that fatty acids are not synthesized and degraded at the same time.

Physiological and Clinical Importance: De novo synthesis of fatty acids is essential for the storage of excess energy in the form of triglycerides and for the synthesis of structural lipids required for cell membranes. Palmitic acid produced by this pathway can be further elongated or desaturated to form other fatty acids as needed by the body. Excessive fatty acid synthesis contributes to metabolic disorders such as obesity, fatty liver and insulin resistance. Therefore, understanding the de novo synthesis of fatty acids provides a biochemical basis for the management of metabolic diseases and the rational use of drugs that target lipid metabolism.

Biological Significance of Cholesterol

Cholesterol is an essential sterol lipid widely distributed in all animal tissues and is a vital component of cell membranes and various biologically important molecules. Although often regarded only in the context of cardiovascular disease, cholesterol plays numerous indispensable physiological roles in the human body. It is synthesized endogenously, mainly in the liver, intestine and other tissues, and is also obtained from dietary sources. The biological significance of cholesterol lies in its structural, metabolic and regulatory functions.

Structural Role in Cell Membranes: One of the most important functions of cholesterol is its role as a structural component of cell membranes. Cholesterol is an integral part of the plasma membrane and intracellular membranes, where it is intercalated between phospholipid molecules. By doing so, cholesterol regulates membrane fluidity and stability. At high temperatures, it reduces excessive membrane fluidity, while at low temperatures, it prevents membrane rigidity. This buffering effect is crucial for maintaining membrane integrity, permeability and proper functioning of membrane-bound proteins, receptors and enzymes. Cholesterol is particularly abundant in membranes of nerve cells and is essential for normal cellular signaling and transport processes.

Precursor of Steroid Hormones: Cholesterol serves as the primary precursor for the synthesis of all steroid hormones in the body. These hormones include glucocorticoids such as cortisol, mineralocorticoids such as aldosterone and sex hormones such as estrogen, progesterone and testosterone. Steroid hormones play vital roles in regulating metabolism, electrolyte balance, immune responses, stress adaptation, growth, development and reproductive functions. Without cholesterol, the synthesis of these essential hormones would not be possible, highlighting its critical role in endocrine regulation.

Formation of Bile Acids and Bile Salts: Cholesterol is the precursor for bile acids and bile salts, which are synthesized in the liver. Bile acids such as cholic acid and chenodeoxycholic acid are converted into bile salts by conjugation with glycine or taurine. Bile salts play a key role in the digestion and absorption of dietary lipids by emulsifying fats in the intestine and facilitating the action of pancreatic lipase. They also aid in the absorption of fat-soluble vitamins A, D, E and K. Thus, cholesterol is indirectly essential for normal lipid digestion and nutritional status.

Precursor of Vitamin D: Cholesterol is also a precursor of vitamin D. In the skin, 7-dehydrocholesterol, a derivative of cholesterol, is converted to cholecalciferol (vitamin D_3) under the influence of ultraviolet rays from sunlight. Vitamin D plays a crucial role in calcium and phosphorus metabolism, bone mineralization and maintenance of skeletal health. Deficiency of vitamin D can lead to disorders such as rickets in children and osteomalacia in adults, emphasizing the importance of cholesterol in vitamin D synthesis.

Role in Myelin Formation and Nervous System Function: Cholesterol is a major component of myelin, the insulating sheath that surrounds nerve fibers. Myelin is essential for the rapid conduction of nerve impulses and proper functioning of the nervous system. High cholesterol content in myelin membranes contributes to their compact structure and electrical insulation properties. Adequate cholesterol levels are therefore necessary for normal brain development, cognitive function and maintenance of neuronal integrity.

Role in Lipoprotein Formation and Lipid Transport: Cholesterol is an important constituent of plasma lipoproteins, including chylomicrons, very low-density lipoproteins, low-density lipoproteins and high-density lipoproteins. These lipoproteins are responsible for the transport of cholesterol and other lipids in the blood to various tissues. Cholesterol transported by lipoproteins is utilized for membrane synthesis, hormone production and other metabolic functions. Proper regulation of cholesterol transport is essential for maintaining lipid homeostasis in the body.

Clinical Significance: While cholesterol is essential for normal physiological functions, excess cholesterol in the blood, particularly in the form of low-density lipoprotein cholesterol, is associated with the development of atherosclerosis and cardiovascular diseases. Deposition of cholesterol in arterial walls leads to plaque formation, which can impair blood flow and increase the risk of heart attack and stroke. Therefore, maintaining a balance between cholesterol synthesis, utilization and excretion is critical for health.

Conversion of Cholesterol into Bile Acids

The conversion of cholesterol into bile acids is one of the most important pathways for the utilization and elimination of cholesterol from the body. Bile acids are synthesized in the liver from cholesterol and play a crucial role in the digestion and absorption of dietary lipids. This process not only facilitates fat digestion but also helps maintain cholesterol homeostasis by preventing excessive accumulation of cholesterol in the body.

Overview and Site of Bile Acid Synthesis: Bile acids are synthesized exclusively in the liver hepatocytes from cholesterol. They are then secreted into bile, stored in the gallbladder and released into the intestine during digestion. The primary bile acids formed in humans are cholic acid and chenodeoxycholic acid. These primary bile acids are further modified in the intestine to form secondary bile acids. The conversion of cholesterol into bile acids is a multistep enzymatic process that takes place mainly in the endoplasmic reticulum, mitochondria and cytosol of liver cells.

Steps in the Conversion of Cholesterol into Primary Bile Acids: The first and rate-limiting step in bile acid synthesis is the hydroxylation of cholesterol at the 7α position. This reaction is catalyzed by the enzyme cholesterol 7α-hydroxylase, which is a microsomal enzyme requiring molecular oxygen, NADPH and cytochrome P450. This step commits cholesterol to bile acid synthesis and is the most important regulatory point in the pathway.

Following 7α-hydroxylation, cholesterol undergoes a series of enzymatic reactions that include further hydroxylation, oxidation and reduction of the steroid nucleus, as well as shortening of the side chain from eight carbon atoms to five carbon atoms. These reactions involve enzymes located in the endoplasmic reticulum and mitochondria. Depending on the pattern of hydroxylation, two primary bile acids are formed. Cholic acid is produced when hydroxyl groups are introduced at the 3α, 7α and 12α positions, while chenodeoxycholic acid is formed when hydroxylation occurs at the 3α and 7α positions only.

Conjugation of Bile Acids: Before secretion into bile, primary bile acids are conjugated with the amino acids glycine or taurine in the liver. This conjugation forms bile salts such as glycocholate, taurocholate, glycochenodeoxycholate and taurochenodeoxycholate. Conjugation increases the water solubility of bile acids and lowers their pKa, making them more effective detergents at the pH of the intestine. Bile salts are the physiologically active forms that participate in lipid digestion.

Formation of Secondary Bile Acids: In the intestine, bile salts undergo further modification by intestinal bacteria. Bacterial enzymes deconjugate and dehydroxylate primary bile acids to form secondary bile acids. Cholic acid is converted into deoxycholic acid, while chenodeoxycholic acid is converted into lithocholic acid. A large portion of bile acids is reabsorbed from the ileum and returned to the liver through the enterohepatic circulation, where they are reused. Only a small fraction is excreted in the feces, representing the major route of cholesterol elimination from the body.

Regulation of Bile Acid Synthesis: The synthesis of bile acids from cholesterol is tightly regulated to maintain cholesterol balance. Cholesterol 7α-hydroxylase is inhibited by bile acids through feedback inhibition. When bile acid levels in the liver increase, the activity of this enzyme decreases, reducing further bile acid synthesis. Conversely, when bile acid levels are low, enzyme activity increases, promoting conversion of cholesterol into bile acids. Hormonal and dietary factors also influence bile acid synthesis.

Biological and Clinical Importance: The conversion of cholesterol into bile acids is biologically significant because it represents the primary mechanism for cholesterol disposal in the body. Bile acids are essential for the emulsification and absorption of dietary fats and fat-soluble vitamins. Impairment of bile acid synthesis or secretion can lead to fat malabsorption and nutritional deficiencies. Clinically, drugs such as bile acid sequestrants lower plasma cholesterol levels by interrupting enterohepatic circulation, thereby increasing the conversion of cholesterol into bile acids. Understanding this pathway is therefore important for pharmacy students in the context of lipid metabolism and pharmacological management of hypercholesterolemia.

Conversion of Cholesterol into Steroid Hormones

The conversion of cholesterol into steroid hormones is a vital biochemical process that forms the basis of endocrine regulation in the human body. Cholesterol acts as the universal precursor for all steroid hormones, which include glucocorticoids, mineralocorticoids and sex hormones. These hormones regulate a wide range of physiological functions such as metabolism, electrolyte balance, stress response, growth, development and reproduction. The synthesis of steroid hormones occurs in specialized endocrine tissues and is tightly regulated to meet the body's needs.

Site and Organs of Steroid Hormone Synthesis: Steroid hormone synthesis takes place mainly in the adrenal cortex, gonads (testes and ovaries) and placenta during pregnancy. The adrenal cortex produces glucocorticoids, mineralocorticoids and adrenal androgens. The testes synthesize androgens such as testosterone, while the ovaries produce estrogens and progesterone. All these hormones are derived from cholesterol, which may be synthesized within the cell or taken up from circulating low-density lipoproteins.

Transport of Cholesterol into Mitochondria: The first step in steroid hormone synthesis is the transport of cholesterol from the cytosol into the mitochondria of steroidogenic cells. This transport is mediated by a specific protein known as the steroidogenic acute regulatory protein (StAR). This step is rate-limiting and highly regulated, as it controls the availability of cholesterol for hormone synthesis. Once inside the mitochondria, cholesterol undergoes enzymatic conversion to initiate steroidogenesis.

Formation of Pregnenolone: The Common Intermediate: The initial and crucial step in the conversion of cholesterol into steroid hormones is the cleavage of the cholesterol side chain to form pregnenolone. This reaction is catalyzed by the mitochondrial enzyme cholesterol desmolase, also known as cytochrome P450 side-chain cleavage enzyme (P450scc). The reaction requires molecular oxygen and NADPH and results in the removal of a six-carbon side chain from cholesterol. Pregnenolone formed in this step serves as the common precursor for all steroid hormones.

Conversion of Pregnenolone into Progesterone: Pregnenolone is transported from the mitochondria to the smooth endoplasmic reticulum, where it is converted into progesterone by the enzyme 3β-hydroxysteroid dehydrogenase. Progesterone is an important steroid hormone itself and also acts as a key intermediate for the synthesis of other steroid hormones. From progesterone, different classes of steroid hormones are produced depending on the tissue-specific enzymes present.

Synthesis of Glucocorticoids: In the adrenal cortex, progesterone undergoes hydroxylation and oxidation reactions to form glucocorticoids, primarily cortisol. These reactions are catalyzed by a series of cytochrome P450 enzymes. Cortisol plays a major role in regulating carbohydrate, protein and lipid metabolism, maintaining blood glucose levels and modulating immune and inflammatory responses. The synthesis of glucocorticoids is regulated by adrenocorticotropic hormone released from the pituitary gland.

Synthesis of Mineralocorticoids: Progesterone also serves as a precursor for mineralocorticoids, mainly aldosterone, which are synthesized in the zona glomerulosa of the adrenal cortex. Aldosterone regulates sodium and potassium balance and helps maintain blood pressure and fluid volume. The synthesis of mineralocorticoids is regulated primarily by the renin-angiotensin-aldosterone system and plasma potassium levels rather than pituitary hormones.

Synthesis of Sex Hormones: In the gonads, pregnenolone and progesterone are converted into sex hormones through tissue-specific pathways. In the testes, progesterone is converted into androgens such as testosterone, which are responsible for male sexual development and maintenance of male reproductive functions. In the ovaries, progesterone and androgens are further converted into estrogens by the enzyme aromatase. Estrogens regulate female reproductive functions, menstrual cycle and secondary sexual characteristics. Progesterone itself plays a crucial role in pregnancy and preparation of the uterus for implantation.

Regulation of Steroid Hormone Synthesis: Steroid hormone synthesis is regulated at multiple levels, including cholesterol availability, StAR protein activity and enzyme expression. Hormones such as adrenocorticotropic hormone, luteinizing hormone and follicle-stimulating hormone stimulate steroidogenesis by increasing cholesterol uptake and enzyme activity. Feedback inhibition by circulating steroid hormones helps maintain hormonal balance.

Biological and Clinical Importance: The conversion of cholesterol into steroid hormones is essential for normal growth, development and homeostasis. Disorders in steroid hormone synthesis can lead to various clinical conditions such as adrenal insufficiency, congenital adrenal hyperplasia, infertility and hormonal imbalances. Understanding this pathway is important for pharmacy students, as many drugs influence steroid hormone synthesis or action, and synthetic steroid hormones are widely used in clinical practice.

Conversion of Cholesterol into Vitamin D

The conversion of cholesterol into vitamin D represents an important metabolic pathway that links lipid metabolism with calcium and phosphorus homeostasis. Vitamin D is a fat-soluble vitamin essential for bone mineralization, normal skeletal growth and maintenance of serum calcium levels. Cholesterol serves as the biochemical precursor for vitamin D synthesis, and this process involves both photochemical and enzymatic reactions occurring in the skin, liver and kidneys.

Precursor of Vitamin D: 7-Dehydrocholesterol: The immediate precursor of vitamin D in the body is 7-dehydrocholesterol, a derivative of cholesterol present in high concentration in the epidermal layers of the skin. 7-Dehydrocholesterol is formed during cholesterol biosynthesis and accumulates in the skin, where it becomes available for conversion into vitamin D under the influence of sunlight.

Photochemical Conversion in the Skin: The first step in vitamin D synthesis occurs in the skin and is a non-enzymatic, photochemical reaction. When the skin is exposed to ultraviolet B radiation from sunlight, 7-dehydrocholesterol absorbs this energy and is converted into previtamin D_3. This compound is thermodynamically unstable and undergoes a spontaneous rearrangement to form cholecalciferol, also known as vitamin D_3. This step is dependent on adequate sunlight exposure and is influenced by factors such as skin pigmentation, age, geographical location and duration of exposure.

Transport of Vitamin D_3 to the Liver: Cholecalciferol formed in the skin enters the bloodstream, where it is transported to the liver bound to a specific carrier protein called vitamin D–binding protein. Dietary vitamin D, if consumed, also enters the circulation and follows the same metabolic pathway. At this stage, vitamin D_3 is biologically inactive and requires further activation through hydroxylation reactions.

Hydroxylation in the Liver: In the liver, cholecalciferol undergoes its first hydroxylation reaction. This reaction is catalyzed by the enzyme vitamin D 25-hydroxylase, which introduces a hydroxyl group at the 25th carbon position of the molecule. The product formed is 25-hydroxycholecalciferol, also known as calcidiol. This is the major circulating form of vitamin D and is used clinically to assess vitamin D status in the body.

Hydroxylation in the Kidney: The second and final activation step occurs in the kidney, where 25-hydroxycholecalciferol is further hydroxylated at the 1α position by the enzyme 1α-hydroxylase. This reaction produces 1,25-dihydroxycholecalciferol, also known as calcitriol, which is the biologically active form of vitamin D. The activity of renal 1α-hydroxylase is tightly regulated by parathyroid hormone, serum calcium and phosphate levels to maintain mineral homeostasis.

Regulation of Vitamin D Synthesis: The synthesis of active vitamin D is finely regulated to prevent toxicity and maintain calcium balance. Low serum calcium and phosphate levels stimulate parathyroid hormone secretion, which in turn enhances renal 1α-hydroxylase activity, increasing calcitriol production. High levels of calcitriol exert negative feedback by inhibiting its own synthesis. Unlike other vitamins, excessive sunlight exposure does not cause vitamin D toxicity because excess previtamin D_3 is converted into inactive photoproducts.

Biological and Clinical Importance: Vitamin D derived from cholesterol plays a crucial role in increasing intestinal absorption of calcium and phosphorus, promoting bone mineralization and maintaining neuromuscular function. Deficiency of vitamin D leads to rickets in children and osteomalacia in adults, while excessive vitamin D can cause hypercalcemia. Understanding the conversion of cholesterol into vitamin D is important for pharmacy students, as vitamin D analogs are used therapeutically in bone disorders, renal disease and certain endocrine conditions.

Disorders of Lipid Metabolism

Disorders of lipid metabolism are a group of conditions that arise due to abnormalities in the digestion, absorption, transport, synthesis or degradation of lipids in the body. Lipids play a central role in energy storage, membrane structure and synthesis of biologically active molecules; therefore, disturbances in lipid metabolism can have wide-ranging effects on health. These disorders may be inherited or acquired and are often associated with significant morbidity, particularly cardiovascular and metabolic complications.

➢ Hypercholesterolemia

Hypercholesterolemia is a metabolic disorder characterized by abnormally elevated levels of cholesterol in the blood, particularly low-density lipoprotein cholesterol. It is one of the most important disorders of lipid metabolism and a major risk factor for the development of atherosclerosis and cardiovascular diseases such as coronary artery disease and stroke. Hypercholesterolemia may arise due to genetic factors, lifestyle habits or as a consequence of other underlying diseases.

Definition and Types of Hypercholesterolemia:

Hypercholesterolemia refers to an increase in total plasma cholesterol concentration above normal levels. It can be classified into primary and secondary types. Primary hypercholesterolemia is caused by inherited genetic defects affecting cholesterol metabolism and lipoprotein clearance. The most common form is familial hypercholesterolemia, which results from mutations in the low-density lipoprotein receptor gene, leading to reduced clearance of LDL cholesterol from the blood.

Secondary hypercholesterolemia develops due to other conditions such as diabetes mellitus, hypothyroidism, nephrotic syndrome, obstructive liver disease and prolonged consumption of a diet rich in saturated fats and cholesterol.

Causes and Risk Factors: The major causes of hypercholesterolemia include increased dietary intake of cholesterol and saturated fats, decreased physical activity and obesity. Genetic factors play a significant role, particularly in familial forms of the disorder. Hormonal imbalances, especially reduced thyroid hormone levels, impair cholesterol metabolism and clearance. Certain drugs such as corticosteroids, thiazide diuretics and oral contraceptives may also contribute to elevated cholesterol levels. Advancing age, smoking and stress further increase the risk of hypercholesterolemia.

Biochemical Basis: The biochemical basis of hypercholesterolemia involves an imbalance between cholesterol synthesis, utilization and excretion. Increased hepatic synthesis of cholesterol, reduced conversion of cholesterol into bile acids and decreased uptake of LDL cholesterol by peripheral tissues all contribute to elevated plasma cholesterol levels. In familial hypercholesterolemia, defective or absent LDL receptors lead to reduced clearance of LDL cholesterol, causing its accumulation in the bloodstream and deposition in tissues.

Clinical Manifestations: Hypercholesterolemia is often asymptomatic in its early stages. With prolonged elevation of cholesterol levels, cholesterol may accumulate in tissues, leading to physical signs such as xanthomas, which are yellowish deposits of cholesterol-rich material in the skin and tendons, and xanthelasma around the eyelids. Long-standing hypercholesterolemia significantly increases the risk of atherosclerosis, resulting in reduced blood flow to vital organs and the development of ischemic heart disease, myocardial infarction and cerebrovascular accidents.

Complications: The most serious complication of hypercholesterolemia is atherosclerosis. Elevated LDL cholesterol promotes deposition of cholesterol in arterial walls, formation of atherosclerotic plaques and narrowing of blood vessels. This process can lead to coronary artery disease, angina pectoris, heart attack, stroke and peripheral vascular disease. Hypercholesterolemia also contributes to the progression of hypertension and may worsen outcomes in patients with diabetes mellitus.

Diagnosis: Diagnosis of hypercholesterolemia is based on lipid profile testing, which includes measurement of total cholesterol, LDL cholesterol, high-density lipoprotein cholesterol and triglycerides. Elevated total and LDL cholesterol levels confirm the diagnosis. Family history, clinical examination and exclusion of secondary causes are important in determining the type of hypercholesterolemia.

Management and Prevention: Management of hypercholesterolemia involves lifestyle modifications and pharmacological therapy. Dietary measures include reducing intake of saturated fats and cholesterol, increasing consumption of dietary fiber and incorporating healthy fats such as polyunsaturated and monounsaturated fatty acids. Regular physical activity and weight reduction help improve lipid profiles. Pharmacological treatment includes the use of statins, which inhibit cholesterol synthesis, bile acid sequestrants, cholesterol absorption inhibitors and PCSK9 inhibitors. Early detection and effective management are essential to prevent cardiovascular complications.

Pharmaceutical Importance: For pharmacy students, understanding hypercholesterolemia is important because it forms the biochemical basis for the rational use of lipid-lowering drugs. Knowledge of cholesterol metabolism, lipoprotein transport and regulatory mechanisms aids in selecting appropriate therapy, monitoring treatment outcomes and counseling patients for long-term disease management.

➤ Atherosclerosis

Atherosclerosis is a chronic, progressive disorder of lipid metabolism characterized by the accumulation of lipids, particularly cholesterol and cholesterol esters, along with fibrous tissue in the walls of medium and large arteries. It is the most important pathological consequence of hypercholesterolemia and a major underlying cause of cardiovascular diseases such as coronary artery disease, myocardial infarction and stroke. Atherosclerosis develops slowly over many years and often remains asymptomatic until significant arterial narrowing or acute vascular events occur.

Etiology and Risk Factors: The development of atherosclerosis is influenced by multiple risk factors. Elevated levels of low-density lipoprotein cholesterol are the most significant biochemical factor contributing to the disease. Other major risk factors include smoking, hypertension, diabetes mellitus, obesity, physical inactivity and increasing age. Genetic predisposition, male gender and family history of premature cardiovascular disease also increase susceptibility. High-density lipoprotein cholesterol has a protective role, and low levels of HDL cholesterol are associated with increased risk of atherosclerosis.

Pathogenesis of Atherosclerosis: The pathogenesis of atherosclerosis begins with injury or dysfunction of the endothelial lining of arteries. This endothelial damage increases permeability to lipoproteins, particularly LDL cholesterol, allowing them to enter the arterial intima. LDL cholesterol undergoes oxidative modification within the arterial wall, becoming oxidized LDL, which plays a central role in plaque formation.

Oxidized LDL stimulates the recruitment of monocytes from the bloodstream into the arterial wall. These monocytes differentiate into macrophages and engulf oxidized LDL through scavenger receptors, forming lipid-laden foam cells. Accumulation of foam cells leads to the formation of fatty streaks, which are the earliest visible lesions of atherosclerosis.

As the disease progresses, smooth muscle cells migrate from the media into the intima and proliferate. These cells synthesize extracellular matrix components such as collagen and elastin, forming a fibrous cap over a lipid-rich necrotic core. This structure is known as an atherosclerotic plaque. Over time, plaques may enlarge, calcify and narrow the arterial lumen, reducing blood flow to tissues.

Role of Lipids and Lipoproteins: Low-density lipoprotein cholesterol is the primary lipid involved in atherogenesis. Elevated LDL levels increase cholesterol deposition in arterial walls. In contrast, high-density lipoprotein cholesterol protects against atherosclerosis by removing excess cholesterol from peripheral tissues and transporting it back to the liver for excretion through a process known as reverse cholesterol transport. An imbalance between LDL and HDL cholesterol significantly influences the development and progression of atherosclerosis.

Clinical Manifestations: The clinical manifestations of atherosclerosis depend on the arteries affected. In coronary arteries, it leads to ischemic heart disease, presenting as angina pectoris or myocardial infarction. In cerebral arteries, atherosclerosis can result in transient ischemic attacks or stroke. In peripheral arteries, it causes peripheral arterial disease, characterized by intermittent claudication, pain, numbness and coldness of extremities. Many patients remain asymptomatic until advanced stages of the disease.

Complications: Atherosclerosis can lead to serious and life-threatening complications. Plaque rupture may trigger the formation of a thrombus, resulting in sudden occlusion of the artery. This can cause acute myocardial infarction, stroke or sudden cardiac death. Chronic narrowing of arteries can lead to tissue ischemia, organ dysfunction and impaired quality of life.

Prevention and Management: Prevention and management of atherosclerosis focus on controlling modifiable risk factors. Lifestyle modifications such as adopting a healthy diet low in saturated fats and cholesterol, regular physical activity, weight management and smoking cessation are essential. Pharmacological therapy includes lipid-lowering agents such as statins, which reduce LDL cholesterol levels and stabilize atherosclerotic plaques. Control of hypertension and diabetes mellitus also plays a crucial role in preventing disease progression.

Pharmaceutical and Clinical Importance: From a pharmaceutical perspective, atherosclerosis is a key target for preventive and therapeutic interventions. Understanding the biochemical and pathological basis of atherosclerosis helps in the rational use of drugs that modify lipid levels, inhibit platelet aggregation and reduce inflammation. For pharmacy students, a thorough knowledge of atherosclerosis provides the foundation for understanding cardiovascular pharmacotherapy and the role of lipid metabolism in disease development.

➢ **Fatty Liver (Hepatic Steatosis)**

Fatty liver, also known as hepatic steatosis, is a metabolic disorder characterized by excessive accumulation of triglycerides within liver cells. It represents an important disorder of lipid metabolism and occurs when the balance between lipid uptake, synthesis, oxidation and export by the liver is disturbed. Fatty liver may be reversible in its early stages, but if persistent, it can progress to more severe liver diseases.

Definition and Types of Fatty Liver: Fatty liver is defined as the presence of lipid droplets, mainly triglycerides, in more than normal amounts within hepatocytes. It can be broadly classified into alcoholic fatty liver and non-alcoholic fatty liver disease. Alcoholic fatty liver develops due to chronic excessive alcohol consumption, whereas non-alcoholic fatty liver disease is associated with metabolic conditions such as obesity, insulin resistance, diabetes mellitus and dyslipidemia. Both forms share common biochemical mechanisms leading to lipid accumulation in the liver.

Causes and Predisposing Factors: The major causes of fatty liver include chronic alcohol intake, obesity, diabetes mellitus, starvation, protein malnutrition and prolonged intake of high-fat or high-carbohydrate diets. Certain drugs such as corticosteroids, methotrexate and some antiretroviral agents can also contribute to fatty liver.

Conditions that impair lipid metabolism, including hypothyroidism and metabolic syndrome, increase the risk of hepatic steatosis.

Biochemical Basis of Fatty Liver: The accumulation of fat in the liver occurs due to an imbalance between the processes that add triglycerides to the liver and those that remove them. Increased mobilization of free fatty acids from adipose tissue leads to excessive delivery of fatty acids to the liver. Enhanced de novo fatty acid synthesis in the liver, particularly in the presence of excess carbohydrates and insulin resistance, further increases triglyceride formation. At the same time, decreased β-oxidation of fatty acids and impaired synthesis or secretion of very low-density lipoproteins reduce the export of triglycerides from the liver. In alcohol-induced fatty liver, increased NADH levels inhibit fatty acid oxidation and promote triglyceride synthesis.

Pathogenesis: In fatty liver, excess triglycerides accumulate as lipid droplets within hepatocytes, causing hepatocellular swelling and enlargement of the liver. Initially, this condition may not cause inflammation or cell death and is often asymptomatic. However, persistent lipid accumulation can lead to oxidative stress, mitochondrial dysfunction and inflammatory responses. Over time, fatty liver may progress to steatohepatitis, characterized by liver inflammation and hepatocyte injury, and may further advance to fibrosis and cirrhosis.

Clinical Features: Fatty liver is often asymptomatic, especially in the early stages. Some patients may experience nonspecific symptoms such as fatigue, malaise and discomfort in the right upper abdomen. Hepatomegaly is a common physical finding. Laboratory investigations may reveal mildly elevated liver enzymes. In advanced cases, symptoms related to liver dysfunction may appear.

Diagnosis: Diagnosis of fatty liver is based on clinical history, laboratory tests and imaging studies. Ultrasound, computed tomography and magnetic resonance imaging can detect fat accumulation in the liver. Liver function tests may show mild elevation of transaminases. In some cases, liver biopsy is required to assess the severity of steatosis and associated inflammation or fibrosis.

Management and Prevention: Management of fatty liver primarily involves addressing the underlying causes. Lifestyle modifications such as weight reduction, dietary changes and regular physical activity are the cornerstone of treatment. Abstinence from alcohol is essential in alcoholic fatty liver disease. Control of diabetes mellitus, dyslipidemia and other metabolic disorders helps prevent disease progression. Pharmacological treatment may be considered in selected cases to improve insulin sensitivity or reduce lipid accumulation.

Clinical and Pharmaceutical Importance: Fatty liver is a growing public health concern due to its association with obesity and metabolic syndrome. From a pharmaceutical perspective, understanding the biochemical mechanisms of fatty liver is important for developing and using drugs that target lipid metabolism and insulin resistance. Early recognition and management are crucial to prevent progression to irreversible liver damage.

- **Obesity**

Obesity is a chronic metabolic disorder characterized by excessive accumulation of body fat resulting from an imbalance between energy intake and energy expenditure. It is one of the most prevalent disorders of lipid metabolism and is closely associated with abnormalities in fat digestion, storage and utilization. Obesity is a major risk factor for several metabolic and cardiovascular diseases and has significant clinical and public health implications.

Definition and Assessment of Obesity: Obesity is defined as an abnormal or excessive fat accumulation that presents a risk to health. It is commonly assessed using the body mass index, which is calculated as weight in kilograms divided by the square of height in meters. A body mass index of 25 to 29.9 kg/m^2 indicates overweight, while a body mass index of 30 kg/m^2 or more is classified as obesity. Excessive accumulation of adipose tissue, particularly in the abdominal region, is associated with higher metabolic risk.

Causes and Predisposing Factors: The primary cause of obesity is a sustained positive energy balance, where caloric intake exceeds energy expenditure. Consumption of energy-dense foods rich in fats and refined carbohydrates, combined with sedentary lifestyle and reduced physical activity, plays a major role. Genetic factors influence appetite regulation, basal metabolic rate and fat storage, predisposing individuals to obesity. Hormonal disturbances, psychological factors, socioeconomic conditions and certain medications such as corticosteroids and antidepressants may also contribute to the development of obesity.

Biochemical Basis of Obesity: At the biochemical level, obesity is associated with increased synthesis and storage of triglycerides in adipose tissue. Excess dietary carbohydrates are converted into fatty acids through de novo lipogenesis and stored as triglycerides. Insulin plays a central role by promoting glucose uptake, fatty acid synthesis and inhibition of lipolysis. In obesity, insulin resistance develops, leading to impaired glucose and lipid metabolism. Increased levels of free fatty acids in circulation further exacerbate metabolic disturbances.

Role of Adipose Tissue and Hormones: Adipose tissue is an active endocrine organ that secretes hormones and cytokines known as adipokines. These include leptin, adiponectin, resistin and inflammatory mediators. Leptin regulates appetite and energy expenditure by acting on the hypothalamus, but in obesity, leptin resistance develops, leading to continued food intake despite high leptin levels. Reduced adiponectin levels impair fatty acid oxidation and insulin sensitivity, contributing to metabolic complications.

Clinical Features and Complications: Obesity is associated with numerous complications affecting multiple organ systems. These include type 2 diabetes mellitus, dyslipidemia, hypertension, atherosclerosis and coronary artery disease. Obesity also increases the risk of fatty liver disease, gallstones, osteoarthritis, sleep apnea and certain cancers.

Psychosocial effects such as reduced quality of life and depression are also common.

Management of Obesity: Management of obesity involves a combination of lifestyle modifications, behavioral therapy and pharmacological interventions. Dietary management focuses on reducing caloric intake while ensuring adequate nutrition. Regular physical activity increases energy expenditure and improves metabolic health. Pharmacological agents may be used to reduce appetite, inhibit fat absorption or improve metabolic parameters in selected patients. In severe cases, bariatric surgery may be considered.

Pharmaceutical and Clinical Importance: For pharmacy students, understanding obesity is essential because it underlies many metabolic disorders and influences drug pharmacokinetics and pharmacodynamics. Obesity alters lipid metabolism, insulin sensitivity and inflammatory status, which can affect drug efficacy and safety. Knowledge of the biochemical basis of obesity aids in the rational selection and counseling of anti-obesity and metabolic drugs.

Chapter-6

Amino Acid Metabolism

Amino acids are the building blocks of proteins and play a central role in numerous metabolic pathways. They are organic compounds containing an amino group (-NH_2), a carboxyl group (-COOH), a hydrogen atom, and a variable side chain (R group) attached to a central α-carbon. Amino acid metabolism encompasses the processes by which amino acids are synthesized, degraded, and utilized for energy production, biosynthesis of nitrogen-containing compounds, and maintenance of nitrogen balance in the body.

Proteins ingested in the diet are first broken down into their constituent amino acids by proteolytic enzymes in the gastrointestinal tract. These amino acids are absorbed into the bloodstream and transported to various tissues, where they serve as substrates for protein synthesis or as precursors for other biomolecules, including neurotransmitters, hormones, heme, purines, and pyrimidines.

Amino acid metabolism can be broadly categorized into **anabolism (synthesis)** and **catabolism (degradation)**. Anabolism refers to the formation of amino acids from simpler molecules, often utilizing intermediates of carbohydrate metabolism or other amino acids. Catabolism involves the breakdown of amino acids to produce energy, intermediates for the tricarboxylic acid (TCA) cycle, or nitrogenous waste, primarily in the form of urea.

Nitrogen metabolism is a crucial aspect of amino acid metabolism. Amino groups removed from amino acids during catabolism are either transferred to other molecules through transamination reactions or converted into ammonia, which is subsequently detoxified via the urea cycle in the liver. Carbon skeletons of amino acids can enter various metabolic pathways, including gluconeogenesis, ketogenesis, or energy production through the TCA cycle, depending on whether the amino acid is glucogenic, ketogenic, or both.

Amino acid metabolism is tightly regulated to maintain homeostasis, support growth, and respond to physiological demands such as fasting, exercise, or disease states. Dysregulation of amino acid metabolism can result in metabolic disorders, accumulation of toxic intermediates, or deficiency states, highlighting its clinical significance.

General Reactions of Amino Acid Metabolism

Amino acid metabolism involves the **breakdown and utilization of amino acids** for energy production, synthesis of biologically important compounds, and maintenance of nitrogen balance in the body. The metabolism of amino acids primarily occurs in the **liver**, although certain reactions can take place in other tissues such as the kidney, muscle, and intestine. The general reactions of amino acid metabolism can be broadly classified into the following categories:

1. Transamination

Transamination is the **transfer of an amino group from an amino acid to an α-keto acid**, usually catalyzed by enzymes called **aminotransferases or transaminases**. This reaction is reversible and plays a central role in amino acid catabolism and synthesis. The most common amino group acceptor is **α-ketoglutarate**, which forms **glutamate**, while the amino acid is converted to its corresponding α-keto acid. For example, the transamination of alanine with α-ketoglutarate produces **pyruvate** and **glutamate**.

Key points:

- Requires **pyridoxal phosphate (PLP)** as a coenzyme derived from vitamin B6.
- Allows interconversion of amino acids and facilitates nitrogen transfer.
- Examples of aminotransferases include **alanine aminotransferase (ALT)** and **aspartate aminotransferase (AST)**.

2. Oxidative Deamination

Oxidative deamination involves the **removal of an amino group from glutamate** in the form of ammonia (NH_3), accompanied by the oxidation of the carbon skeleton. This reaction is catalyzed by **glutamate dehydrogenase** and occurs mainly in the liver mitochondria. The reaction produces **α-ketoglutarate** and **ammonia**, which enters the **urea cycle** for excretion.

Key points:

- Provides free ammonia for urea synthesis.
- Links amino acid catabolism with energy metabolism.
- Reversible under certain conditions to facilitate amino acid synthesis.

3. Deamination of Serine and Threonine

Certain amino acids, such as **serine and threonine,** undergo direct deamination without prior transamination. Enzymes like **serine dehydratase** and **threonine dehydratase** catalyze these reactions, producing **pyruvate** and **α-ketobutyrate**, respectively, along with ammonia.

4. Ureagenesis

The ammonia generated from amino acid catabolism is toxic and must be detoxified. In the **liver**, ammonia combines with carbon dioxide to form **urea** via the **urea cycle (ornithine cycle)**. Ureagenesis ensures safe excretion of nitrogen through urine and maintains **nitrogen balance**.

5. Decarboxylation

Amino acids can undergo decarboxylation, in which the **carboxyl group (-COOH) is removed**, forming **biologically active amines** such as **histamine, serotonin, and dopamine**. This reaction is catalyzed by **decarboxylases**, which also require **pyridoxal phosphate (PLP)** as a cofactor.

6. Side-Chain Reactions

Amino acids with specific functional groups undergo **modification of their side chains** to form key metabolites. For example:

- **Methionine** undergoes transmethylation to generate **S-adenosylmethionine (SAM)**, a universal methyl donor.
- **Phenylalanine** is hydroxylated to **tyrosine**, which serves as a precursor for catecholamines and melanin.
- **Tryptophan** is converted to **niacin (vitamin B3)** and serotonin.

7. Carbon Skeleton Oxidation

After removal of the amino group, the remaining **carbon skeletons (α-keto acids)** enter central metabolic pathways for energy production or biosynthesis. Depending on the fate of the carbon skeleton, amino acids are classified as:

- **Glucogenic** – can be converted to glucose via gluconeogenesis. Examples: alanine, serine.
- **Ketogenic** – converted to acetyl-CoA or acetoacetate, contributing to ketone body formation. Examples: leucine, lysine.
- **Both glucogenic and ketogenic** – e.g., isoleucine, phenylalanine, tyrosine.

➢ **Transamination**

Transamination is a fundamental reaction in amino acid metabolism that involves the **transfer of an amino group ($-NH_2$) from an amino acid to an α-keto acid**, resulting in the formation of a **new amino acid** and a **new α-keto acid**. This reaction is **reversible** and plays a central role in both the **catabolism and biosynthesis of amino acids**, as well as in the **transfer of nitrogen** within the body.

Mechanism of Transamination: Transamination reactions are catalyzed by enzymes called **aminotransferases or transaminases**, and they require **pyridoxal phosphate (PLP)**, a coenzyme derived from **vitamin B6**. The reaction occurs in two main steps:

- The amino group from the donor amino acid is temporarily transferred to PLP, forming a **pyridoxamine phosphate intermediate**.
- The amino group is then transferred from pyridoxamine phosphate to the acceptor α-keto acid, forming a new amino acid and regenerating

PLP.

Common Transaminase Reactions: Several aminotransferases catalyze specific transamination reactions:

- **Alanine aminotransferase (ALT or GPT)**: Catalyzes the reaction between **alanine** and **α-ketoglutarate**, forming **pyruvate** and **glutamate**.
- **Aspartate aminotransferase (AST or GOT)**: Catalyzes the reaction between **aspartate** and **α-ketoglutarate**, forming **oxaloacetate** and **glutamate**.

These reactions are crucial for **nitrogen transport** from peripheral tissues to the liver. For example, amino groups from muscle amino acids are transferred to α-ketoglutarate to form glutamate, which can then enter the **urea cycle** for safe nitrogen excretion.

Physiological Significance of Transamination: Transamination reactions are important for several reasons:

- **Amino acid biosynthesis**: Allows the synthesis of non-essential amino acids from corresponding α-keto acids.
- **Nitrogen metabolism**: Facilitates the safe transport of nitrogen between tissues.
- **Energy metabolism**: The α-keto acids formed can enter the **citric acid cycle** to produce energy.
- **Detoxification**: Helps in channeling nitrogen for urea formation, preventing ammonia accumulation.

Clinical Relevance: The activity of aminotransferases, especially **ALT and AST**, is used as a **diagnostic marker for liver function**. Elevated levels in the blood indicate **liver damage** or hepatocellular injury, as these enzymes are released into circulation when hepatocytes are damaged.

➢ Deamination

Deamination is a metabolic process in which the **amino group ($-NH_2$) of an amino acid is removed**, resulting in the formation of a **free**

ammonia (NH_3 or NH_4^+) and a corresponding **α-keto acid**. This reaction is crucial for **amino acid catabolism**, as it allows the **carbon skeleton** to be used for energy production or as precursors for other metabolic pathways, while the nitrogen is safely disposed of through the **urea cycle**. Deamination can occur through **oxidative or non-oxidative pathways**.

Oxidative Deamination: Oxidative deamination is the **removal of an amino group from glutamate** with the concurrent oxidation of the carbon skeleton. This reaction is catalyzed by the enzyme **glutamate dehydrogenase**, which is located in the **mitochondria of liver cells**. The general reaction can be represented as:

Glutamate + NAD^+ (or $NADP^+$) + H_2O → α-Ketoglutarate + NH_4^+ + NADH (or NADPH) + H^+

Key features:

- The amino group is released as **ammonia**, which is toxic and enters the **urea cycle** for excretion.
- The α-ketoglutarate produced can re-enter the **citric acid cycle** for energy production.
- This reaction is **reversible**, allowing amino acid synthesis when needed.

Non-Oxidative or Direct Deamination: Certain amino acids undergo direct deamination without prior transamination. Examples include **serine** and **threonine**:

- **Serine dehydratase** catalyzes the conversion of **serine → pyruvate + NH_4^+**.
- **Threonine dehydratase** catalyzes the conversion of **threonine → α-ketobutyrate + NH_4^+**.

These reactions allow the carbon skeletons of serine and threonine to enter central metabolic pathways, such as **gluconeogenesis or ketogenesis**, while the ammonia produced is channeled into **urea formation**.

Physiological Significance of Deamination: Deamination plays several important roles:

- Provides **free ammonia** for urea synthesis, preventing **hyperammonemia**, which is toxic to the nervous system.
- Generates **α-keto acids**, which serve as substrates for **energy production**, gluconeogenesis, or ketone body formation.
- Maintains **nitrogen balance** by enabling excretion of excess nitrogen.

Clinical Relevance

- Defects in deamination enzymes, particularly **glutamate dehydrogenase**, can result in abnormal **amino acid and nitrogen metabolism**, potentially leading to **hyperammonemia**.
- Monitoring ammonia levels in blood can help in diagnosing **liver dysfunction** or **urea cycle disorders**.

➢ Decarboxylation

Decarboxylation is a metabolic reaction in which the **carboxyl group (-COOH) of an amino acid is removed** as **carbon dioxide (CO_2)**, resulting in the formation of **biologically active amines**. This reaction is catalyzed by enzymes called **amino acid decarboxylases** and requires **pyridoxal phosphate (PLP)**, a coenzyme derived from **vitamin B6**, for activity. Decarboxylation plays a key role in the **synthesis of neurotransmitters and other bioactive molecules**.

Mechanism of Decarboxylation: The general mechanism involves the binding of the amino acid to **PLP**, which stabilizes the carbanion intermediate formed after the removal of the carboxyl group. The reaction releases **CO_2** and produces the corresponding **amine**.

Examples of Amino Acid Decarboxylation: Different amino acids undergo decarboxylation to produce important biological amines:

- **Histidine → Histamine**: Catalyzed by **histidine decarboxylase**; histamine is involved in **inflammatory responses, gastric acid secretion, and neurotransmission**.
- **Glutamate → γ-Aminobutyric Acid (GABA)**: Catalyzed by

glutamate decarboxylase; GABA is the primary **inhibitory neurotransmitter** in the central nervous system.

- **Tyrosine → Dopamine**: Tyrosine is first hydroxylated to **L-DOPA**, which is then decarboxylated by **aromatic L-amino acid decarboxylase** to form **dopamine**, a catecholamine neurotransmitter.
- **Tryptophan → Serotonin (5-hydroxytryptamine, 5-HT)**: Tryptophan is first hydroxylated to **5-hydroxytryptophan** and then decarboxylated to **serotonin**, which regulates **mood, sleep, and appetite**.
- **Ornithine → Putrescine**: Part of **polyamine synthesis**, which is important for **cell growth and differentiation**.

Physiological Significance of Decarboxylation

- Produces **neurotransmitters** such as dopamine, serotonin, and GABA, essential for **nervous system function**.
- Generates **histamine**, which is crucial in **immune responses** and **gastric acid secretion**.
- Contributes to the synthesis of **polyamines**, which are vital for **cell growth, proliferation, and tissue repair**.

Clinical Relevance

- Deficiency of **vitamin B6 (pyridoxine)** can impair decarboxylation reactions, leading to **neurological symptoms**, including seizures, irritability, and peripheral neuropathy.
- Overproduction of decarboxylation products can contribute to **pathological conditions**, such as excessive histamine causing **allergic reactions** or altered neurotransmitter levels affecting **mood and behavior**.

Urea Cycle (Ornithine Cycle)

The **urea cycle**, also known as the **ornithine cycle**, is the primary metabolic pathway by which the **body eliminates excess nitrogen** generated from amino acid catabolism. Since **ammonia (NH_3)** is highly toxic, particularly to the nervous system, the liver converts it into **urea**, a less toxic compound that is excreted in the urine. This cycle is central to **nitrogen balance** in humans and is closely linked with **amino acid metabolism**.

Location and Overview

- The urea cycle occurs **primarily in the liver**, with minor contributions from the kidney.
- It involves both **mitochondrial** and **cytosolic** enzymes.
- The cycle starts with **ammonia,** which is generated by **oxidative deamination of glutamate**, and **aspartate**, which provides a second nitrogen atom.
- Carbon dioxide (CO_2) provides the carbon atom for urea formation.

Steps of the Urea Cycle

Step 1: Formation of Carbamoyl Phosphate

- Enzyme: **Carbamoyl phosphate synthetase I (CPS I)**
- Location: Mitochondria
- Reaction: **NH_4^+ + CO_2 + 2 ATP → Carbamoyl phosphate + 2 ADP + Pi**
- Significance: This is the **rate-limiting step** of the urea cycle and requires **N-acetylglutamate** as an allosteric activator.

Step 2: Formation of Citrulline

- Enzyme: **Ornithine transcarbamylase (OTC)**
- Reaction: **Carbamoyl phosphate + Ornithine → Citrulline**
- Citrulline is transported from the mitochondria to the cytosol.

Step 3: Formation of Argininosuccinate

- Enzyme: **Argininosuccinate synthetase**
- Reaction: **Citrulline + Aspartate + ATP → Argininosuccinate + AMP + PPi**
- Aspartate provides the **second nitrogen** for urea formation.

Step 4: Formation of Arginine

- Enzyme: **Argininosuccinate lyase**
- Reaction: **Argininosuccinate → Arginine + Fumarate**

- Fumarate can enter the **citric acid cycle** or be converted to malate and then oxaloacetate for gluconeogenesis.

Step 5: Formation of Urea

- Enzyme: **Arginase**
- Reaction: **Arginine + H_2O → Urea + Ornithine**
- Ornithine is transported back into the mitochondria to continue the cycle.
- Urea is transported to the kidneys for excretion in urine.

Regulation of the Urea Cycle

- **Substrate availability**: High levels of ammonia and amino acids stimulate the cycle.
- **Allosteric activation**: **N-acetylglutamate** activates CPS I.
- **Hormonal regulation**: Glucagon increases the synthesis of urea cycle enzymes during protein-rich diets.

Disorders of the Urea Cycle

Urea cycle disorders (UCDs) are **genetic defects in one of the enzymes** of the cycle, leading to **hyperammonemia** and **toxic accumulation of nitrogenous compounds**. Common disorders include:

a. Carbamoyl Phosphate Synthetase I (CPS I) Deficiency

- Autosomal recessive disorder.
- Leads to **accumulation of ammonia** in the blood.
- Symptoms: Lethargy, vomiting, seizures, developmental delay, and in severe cases, coma.

b. Ornithine Transcarbamylase (OTC) Deficiency

- X-linked recessive disorder, most common UCD.
- Accumulation of **carbamoyl phosphate,** which is converted to **orotic acid,** causing **orotic aciduria.**
- Symptoms: Hyperammonemia, vomiting, lethargy, and neurological deficits.

c. Argininosuccinate Synthetase (Citrullinemia) Deficiency

- Autosomal recessive.
- Citrulline accumulates in the blood.

- Symptoms: Hyperammonemia, poor feeding, vomiting, and growth retardation.

d. Argininosuccinate Lyase Deficiency

- Leads to **argininosuccinic aciduria**.
- Symptoms: Hyperammonemia, developmental delay, liver dysfunction, and brittle hair.

e. Arginase Deficiency

- Rare, autosomal recessive disorder.
- Hyperargininemia occurs rather than severe hyperammonemia.
- Symptoms: Progressive spasticity, growth retardation, and neurological deficits.

Clinical Significance of Urea Cycle Disorders

- Hyperammonemia is **neurotoxic**, leading to cerebral edema, intellectual disability, and in severe cases, death if untreated.
- Early diagnosis through **blood ammonia levels, plasma amino acid analysis, and genetic testing** is critical.
- Treatment includes **low-protein diet, ammonia scavenger drugs**, supplementation with **arginine or citrulline**, and in severe cases, **liver transplantation**.

Catabolism of Phenylalanine

Phenylalanine is an **essential amino acid,** obtained from the diet. Its catabolism primarily occurs in the **liver** and involves the following steps:

Step 1: Hydroxylation to Tyrosine

- Enzyme: **Phenylalanine hydroxylase (PAH)**
- Cofactor: **Tetrahydrobiopterin (BH_4)**
- Reaction: **Phenylalanine + O_2 + BH_4 → Tyrosine + H_2O + BH_2**
- Significance: This is the **rate-limiting step** of phenylalanine catabolism. It converts phenylalanine into tyrosine, which then serves as a substrate for further degradation.

Step 2: Transamination of Tyrosine

- Enzyme: **Tyrosine aminotransferase**
- Reaction: **Tyrosine + α-ketoglutarate → p-**

Hydroxyphenylpyruvate + Glutamate

- Significance: Converts tyrosine into **p-hydroxyphenylpyruvate**, linking amino acid catabolism to the **citric acid cycle** via α-keto acids.

Catabolism of Tyrosine

Tyrosine undergoes a series of reactions to be converted into **fumarate** (a citric acid cycle intermediate) and **acetoacetate** (a ketogenic substrate):

Step 1: Conversion to p-Hydroxyphenylpyruvate

- As above, catalyzed by **tyrosine aminotransferase.**

Step 2: Formation of Homogentisate

- Enzyme: **p-Hydroxyphenylpyruvate dioxygenase**
- Reaction: **p-Hydroxyphenylpyruvate → Homogentisate**
- Significance: Prepares the aromatic ring for cleavage in subsequent steps.

Step 3: Conversion to Maleylacetoacetate

- Enzyme: **Homogentisate dioxygenase**
- Reaction: **Homogentisate → Maleylacetoacetate**
- Significance: Oxidative cleavage of the aromatic ring facilitates further breakdown.

Step 4: Isomerization to Fumarylacetoacetate

- Enzyme: **Maleylacetoacetate isomerase**
- Reaction: **Maleylacetoacetate → Fumarylacetoacetate**
- Significance: Prepares the molecule for hydrolysis to usable metabolic intermediates.

Step 5: Hydrolysis to Fumarate and Acetoacetate

- Enzyme: **Fumarylacetoacetate hydrolase**
- Reaction: **Fumarylacetoacetate → Fumarate + Acetoacetate**
- Significance:
  - **Fumarate** enters the **citric acid cycle** for energy production.
  - **Acetoacetate** is a **ketogenic substrate**, contributing to **ketone body formation.**

Metabolic Disorders of Phenylalanine and Tyrosine

Defects in the catabolic pathways of **phenylalanine and tyrosine** result in the accumulation of toxic intermediates, leading to several **inborn errors of metabolism**. These disorders are inherited, mostly as **autosomal recessive traits**, and have **distinct biochemical and clinical features.**

1. Phenylketonuria (PKU)

- **Cause:** Deficiency of **phenylalanine hydroxylase (PAH)** or its cofactor **tetrahydrobiopterin (BH_4)**.
- **Biochemical Consequence:** Accumulation of **phenylalanine** and its metabolites (phenylpyruvate, phenylacetate, phenyllactate) in blood and urine.
- **Clinical Features**
    - Intellectual disability if untreated
    - Microcephaly and developmental delay
    - Fair skin and hair due to reduced melanin formation
    - Musty odor of urine caused by phenylketones
- **Treatment**
    - Lifelong **low-phenylalanine diet**
    - Supplementation with **tyrosine**, which becomes conditionally essential

2. Albinism

- **Cause:** Deficiency of **tyrosinase**, the enzyme responsible for converting **tyrosine to melanin.**
- **Biochemical Consequence:** Reduced or absent **melanin production**.
- **Clinical Features:**
    - Hypopigmentation of skin, hair, and eyes
    - Visual defects including nystagmus, photophobia, and reduced visual acuity
    - Increased susceptibility to **sunburn and skin cancer**
- **Treatment**

- o Protection from sunlight and ultraviolet exposure
- o Use of **visual aids** for eye defects

3. Alkaptonuria

- **Cause:** Deficiency of **homogentisate dioxygenase**, an enzyme in tyrosine catabolism.
- **Biochemical Consequence:** Accumulation of **homogentisic acid**, which oxidizes to a dark pigment in connective tissues and urine.
- **Clinical Features**
  - o **Dark-colored urine** upon standing
  - o **Ochronosis**: bluish-black pigmentation of cartilage, sclera, and skin
  - o Early-onset **arthritis**, particularly in the spine and large joints
- **Treatment**
  - o Low-protein diet to reduce phenylalanine and tyrosine intake
  - o **Vitamin C supplementation** may slow pigment deposition
  - o Symptomatic management of joint degeneration

4. Tyrosinemia

Tyrosinemia refers to a group of disorders resulting from defects in **enzymes downstream in tyrosine catabolism**.

- **Type I (Hepatorenal Tyrosinemia)**
  - o **Enzyme Deficiency:** Fumarylacetoacetate hydrolase
  - o **Consequence:** Accumulation of fumarylacetoacetate and succinylacetone
  - o **Clinical Features:** Liver failure, renal tubular dysfunction, rickets, cabbage-like odor, neurological crises
  - o **Treatment:** NTBC (nitisinone) therapy, low-tyrosine/phenylalanine diet, liver transplantation if severe
- **Type II (Richner-Hanhart Syndrome)**
  - o **Enzyme Deficiency:** Tyrosine aminotransferase
  - o **Consequence:** Accumulation of tyrosine
  - o **Clinical Features:** Painful keratopathy, thickened palms and soles, intellectual impairment

- **Treatment:** Low-tyrosine and low-phenylalanine diet
- **Type III**
  - **Enzyme Deficiency:** p-Hydroxyphenylpyruvate dioxygenase
  - **Consequence:** Elevated tyrosine levels
  - **Clinical Features:** Neurological symptoms including seizures and cognitive deficits
  - **Treatment:** Dietary restriction of tyrosine and phenylalanine

Synthesis and Significance of Biological Substances

Amino acids are the **building blocks of proteins**, but they also serve as precursors for a wide variety of **bioactive molecules**, including neurotransmitters, hormones, and signaling molecules. These substances regulate critical physiological functions such as **nervous system activity, circadian rhythm, cardiovascular function, metabolism, and immune responses**. The following is a detailed account of the **synthesis pathways, cofactors, regulation, and physiological significance** of key biogenic amines derived from amino acids.

1. Serotonin (5-Hydroxytryptamine, 5-HT)

Synthesis Pathway

- **Precursor:** Tryptophan (essential amino acid)
- **Step 1: Hydroxylation** – Tryptophan is converted to **5-hydroxytryptophan (5-HTP)** by the enzyme **tryptophan hydroxylase**.
  - **Cofactors: Tetrahydrobiopterin (BH_4)**, oxygen, and ferrous ion (Fe^{2+})
  - **Significance:** This is the **rate-limiting step**; regulation occurs via feedback inhibition by serotonin.
- **Step 2: Decarboxylation** – 5-HTP is decarboxylated by **aromatic L-amino acid decarboxylase (PLP-dependent)** to form **serotonin (5-HT)**.
  - **Cofactor:** Pyridoxal phosphate (PLP, vitamin B6 derivative)

Physiological Significance

- **Central Nervous System (CNS):** Acts as a neurotransmitter modulating **mood, anxiety, sleep, appetite, cognition, and pain perception**.

- **Gastrointestinal Tract:** Regulates **intestinal motility** and **secretion**; most serotonin in the body (~90%) is found in the gut.
- **Cardiovascular System:** Influences **vascular tone and platelet aggregation**.
- **Precursor for Melatonin:** Serotonin is converted into **melatonin** in the pineal gland, linking neurotransmitter function with circadian regulation.

Clinical Significance

- **Deficiency:** Associated with **depression, anxiety, insomnia, and irritable bowel syndrome**.
- **Excess:** Can lead to **serotonin syndrome**, especially when taking serotonin-elevating drugs.

2. Melatonin

Synthesis Pathway

- **Precursor:** Serotonin (5-HT)
- **Step 1: N-Acetylation** – Serotonin is acetylated by **serotonin N-acetyltransferase (arylalkylamine N-acetyltransferase)** to form **N-acetylserotonin**.
    - **Cofactor:** Acetyl-CoA
    - **Regulation:** This enzyme is **rate-limiting** and controlled by **light exposure** via the suprachiasmatic nucleus of the hypothalamus.
- **Step 2: O-Methylation** – N-acetylserotonin is methylated by **hydroxyindole-O-methyltransferase (HIOMT)** using **S-adenosylmethionine (SAM)** as the methyl donor to produce **melatonin**.

Physiological Significance

- **Circadian Rhythm:** Regulates **sleep-wake cycles** by signaling darkness to the body.
- **Antioxidant:** Scavenges free radicals, reducing oxidative stress.
- **Immune System:** Enhances **immune function** and modulates inflammatory responses.

- **Reproductive System:** Influences **seasonal reproductive cycles** in animals.

Clinical Significance

- **Deficiency:** Sleep disorders, jet lag, and circadian rhythm disturbances.
- **Therapeutic Use:** Exogenous melatonin supplements for **insomnia, shift work disorder, and jet lag.**

3. Dopamine

Synthesis Pathway

- **Precursor:** Tyrosine (non-essential amino acid, synthesized from phenylalanine)
- **Step 1: Hydroxylation** – Tyrosine is converted into **L-DOPA** by **tyrosine hydroxylase**, the **rate-limiting step**.
    - **Cofactors:** Tetrahydrobiopterin (BH_4), O_2, Fe^{2+}
    - **Regulation:** Feedback inhibition by dopamine
- **Step 2: Decarboxylation** – L-DOPA is converted into **dopamine** by **aromatic L-amino acid decarboxylase (PLP-dependent)**.

Physiological Significance

- **CNS:** Regulates **motor control, emotion, motivation, and reward pathways.**
- **Endocrine:** Modulates **prolactin secretion** from the pituitary gland.
- **Renal Function:** Promotes **natriuresis** and **renal blood flow**.
- **Precursor for Catecholamines:** Dopamine is converted to **noradrenaline** and subsequently **adrenaline.**

Clinical Significance

- **Deficiency:** Leads to **Parkinson's disease**, characterized by tremors, rigidity, and bradykinesia.
- **Excess:** Can contribute to **schizophrenia** and psychotic disorders.

4. Noradrenaline (Norepinephrine)

Synthesis Pathway

- **Precursor:** Dopamine

- **Enzyme: Dopamine β-hydroxylase**
- **Reaction:** Dopamine + O_2 + ascorbate → Noradrenaline + dehydroascorbate
- **Location:** Sympathetic nerve terminals and adrenal medulla vesicles

Physiological Significance

- **Sympathetic Nervous System:** Main neurotransmitter mediating **fight-or-flight response.**
- **Cardiovascular Effects:** Increases **heart rate, cardiac contractility, and vascular tone**, thereby elevating blood pressure.
- **Metabolic Effects:** Stimulates **glycogenolysis, lipolysis,** and energy mobilization.
- **CNS:** Enhances **alertness, attention, and arousal**.

Clinical Significance

- **Deficiency:** Can cause **orthostatic hypotension and reduced stress response.**
- **Excess:** Leads to **hypertension, anxiety, and palpitations**.

5. Adrenaline (Epinephrine)

Synthesis Pathway

- **Precursor:** Noradrenaline
- **Enzyme: Phenylethanolamine N-methyltransferase (PNMT)**
- **Reaction:** Noradrenaline + S-adenosylmethionine (SAM) → Adrenaline + S-adenosylhomocysteine
- **Location:** Adrenal medulla
- **Regulation:** Controlled by sympathetic stimulation and cortisol levels from the adrenal cortex.

Physiological Significance

- **Fight-or-Flight Hormone:** Prepares the body for **stress and emergency response.**
- **Cardiovascular:** Increases **heart rate, cardiac output, and blood pressure.**
- **Metabolism:** Promotes **glycogenolysis, gluconeogenesis,**

lipolysis, and increases **blood glucose and free fatty acids.**

- **Respiration:** Causes **bronchodilation**, enhancing oxygen supply to tissues.

Clinical Significance

- **Deficiency:** Rare; may impair stress response.
- **Excess:** Seen in **pheochromocytoma,** causing **hypertension, tachycardia, and sweating.**

Catabolism of Heme

Heme catabolism occurs primarily in **reticuloendothelial cells of the spleen, liver, and bone marrow**, where **senescent red blood cells (RBCs)** are degraded. The pathway involves several enzymatic steps:

Step 1: Formation of Biliverdin

- **Enzyme:** Heme oxygenase
- **Cofactors:** NADPH, O_2
- **Reaction:** Heme + 3 O_2 + NADPH → Biliverdin + Fe^{2+} + CO + $NADP^+$
- **Significance:**
  - Releases **ferrous iron (Fe^{2+})** for recycling
  - Produces **carbon monoxide (CO)**, which acts as a signaling molecule

Step 2: Conversion of Biliverdin to Bilirubin

- **Enzyme:** Biliverdin reductase
- **Cofactor:** NADPH
- **Reaction:** Biliverdin + NADPH + H^+ → Bilirubin (unconjugated) + $NADP^+$
- **Significance:** Bilirubin is **lipid-soluble** and transported in blood bound to **albumin** to the liver

Step 3: Hepatic Conjugation of Bilirubin

- **Location:** Hepatocytes
- **Enzyme:** UDP-glucuronyltransferase
- **Reaction:** Bilirubin + 2 UDP-glucuronic acid → Bilirubin diglucuronide (conjugated bilirubin)

- **Significance:** Conjugation renders bilirubin **water-soluble,** allowing **excretion in bile**

Step 4: Excretion in Bile and Conversion in Intestine

- Conjugated bilirubin is secreted into bile → intestine
- In the intestine, **bacterial enzymes** convert it to **urobilinogen**
- **Fates of urobilinogen:**
  - Part oxidized to **stercobilin** → excreted in feces (gives brown color)
  - Part reabsorbed into blood → excreted by kidney as **urobilin**

Hyperbilirubinemia

It is an **elevated level of bilirubin** in the blood above the normal range (≈1 mg/dL). It can be **conjugated (direct) or unconjugated (indirect)**, depending on the underlying defect.

Causes of Hyperbilirubinemia

A. Pre-Hepatic (Excess Production of Bilirubin)

- **Mechanism:** Increased breakdown of RBCs (hemolysis) → more **unconjugated bilirubin** than liver can conjugate
- **Examples:** Hemolytic anemia, sickle cell anemia, transfusion reactions

B. Hepatic (Impaired Conjugation or Hepatocellular Dysfunction)

- **Mechanism:** Liver cells cannot conjugate or excrete bilirubin efficiently
- **Causes:**
  - **Neonatal jaundice:** Immature UDP-glucuronyltransferase
  - **Gilbert's syndrome:** Mild decrease in enzyme activity
  - **Crigler-Najjar syndrome:** Severe deficiency of UDP-glucuronyltransferase
  - **Hepatitis, cirrhosis:** Hepatocellular damage

C. Post-Hepatic (Obstruction of Bile Flow)

- **Mechanism:** Conjugated bilirubin cannot reach intestine → regurgitates into blood
- **Causes:** Gallstones, tumors of bile duct or pancreas, cholestasis

Jaundice

It is a yellow discoloration of the **skin, sclera, and mucous membranes** due to **elevated bilirubin** in blood and tissues.

Types of Jaundice

1. Pre-Hepatic Jaundice

- **Bilirubin Type:** Predominantly **unconjugated**
- **Causes:** Hemolysis, ineffective erythropoiesis
- **Features:** Dark urine usually absent (unconjugated bilirubin is not water-soluble)

2. Hepatic Jaundice

- **Bilirubin Type:** Mixed **unconjugated and conjugated**
- **Causes:** Viral hepatitis, alcoholic liver disease, cirrhosis
- **Features:** Dark urine (due to conjugated bilirubin), pale stools, hepatomegaly

3. Post-Hepatic (Obstructive) Jaundice

- **Bilirubin Type:** Predominantly **conjugated**
- **Causes:** Gallstones, biliary atresia, pancreatic tumor
- **Features:** Dark urine, pale stools, pruritus, possible abdominal pain

Chapter-7

Nucleic Acid Metabolism and Genetic Information Transfer

Biosynthesis of Purine and Pyrimidine Nucleotides

Nucleotides are organic molecules consisting of a nitrogenous base, a pentose sugar (ribose or deoxyribose), and one or more phosphate groups. They are essential for the synthesis of nucleic acids (DNA and RNA), serve as energy carriers (ATP, GTP), and act as cofactors in enzymatic reactions (NAD^+, FAD). Nucleotide biosynthesis occurs through two main pathways: **de novo synthesis**, which creates nucleotides from simple precursors, and **salvage pathways**, which recycle free bases or nucleosides.

The **de novo pathways** for purines and pyrimidines differ in the order of assembly:

- **Purines:** the purine ring is built **on ribose** from PRPP.
- **Pyrimidines:** the pyrimidine ring is **assembled first**, then attached to ribose from PRPP.

A. Biosynthesis of Purine Nucleotides

Purine nucleotides include **adenine (A) and guanine (G)**. The nucleotide forms are **IMP (inosine monophosphate), AMP (adenosine monophosphate), and GMP (guanosine monophosphate)**. Purine biosynthesis is a **highly regulated, multi-step process** mainly occurring in the **liver cytosol**.

1. Formation of PRPP (Phosphoribosyl Pyrophosphate)

- **Substrate:** Ribose-5-phosphate (from the pentose phosphate pathway)
- **Enzyme:** PRPP synthetase
- **Cofactor:** ATP (provides energy)
- **Reaction:**

Ribose-5-phosphate + ATP → PRPP + AMP

- **Significance:** PRPP is an activated ribose donor that serves as the backbone for purine ring assembly.

2. Formation of 5-Phosphoribosylamine (PRPP Amidotransferase Reaction)

- **Substrates:** PRPP + Glutamine (provides nitrogen for N9 position of purine)
- **Enzyme:** Glutamine-PRPP amidotransferase (rate-limiting)
- **Reaction:**

PRPP + Glutamine → 5-Phosphoribosylamine + Glutamate + PPi

- **Regulation**
  - Inhibited by **IMP, AMP, GMP** (feedback inhibition)
  - Activated by **PRPP** (substrate availability)
- **Significance:** Commits the pathway to purine biosynthesis.

3. Stepwise Assembly of the Purine Ring (IMP Formation)

The purine ring is **built atom by atom on the ribose sugar** using various donors: glycine, glutamine, aspartate, formate, and CO_2. The intermediates are:

1. **GAR (Glycinamide ribonucleotide)**
   - Formed by adding **glycine** to 5-phosphoribosylamine.
   - Glycine contributes **C4, C5,** N7 of the purine ring.
   - **Enzyme:** GAR synthetase (requires ATP).
2. **FGAR (Formylglycinamide ribonucleotide)**
   - **Formyl group** added from **N10-formyl tetrahydrofolate**.
   - **Enzyme:** GAR transformylase
3. **FGAM (Formylglycinamidine ribonucleotide)**
   - **Nitrogen** from glutamine is added.
   - **Enzyme:** FGAM synthetase (ATP-dependent)
4. **AIR (5-Aminoimidazole ribonucleotide)**
   - Cyclization forms the **imidazole ring.**
   - **Enzyme:** AIR synthetase
5. **CAIR (Carboxyaminoimidazole ribonucleotide)**

- o **Carbon dioxide** added.
- o **Enzyme:** AIR carboxylase

6. **SAICAR(Succinylaminoimidazolecarboxamide ribonucleotide)**

- o Aspartate contributes **C and N**.
- o **Enzyme:** SAICAR synthetase

7. **AICAR (Aminoimidazolecarboxamide ribonucleotide)**

- o Fumarate eliminated from SAICAR.
- o **Enzyme:** Adenylosuccinate lyase

8. **FAICAR (Formyl-AICAR)**

- o Formyl group added from N10-formyl tetrahydrofolate.
- o **Enzyme:** AICAR transformylase

9. **IMP (Inosine monophosphate)**

- o Cyclization completes the **purine ring**.
- o IMP is the **branch point** for AMP and GMP synthesis.

4. Conversion of IMP to AMP and GMP

- **AMP synthesis:** IMP + Aspartate + GTP → Adenylosuccinate → AMP + Fumarate
  - o **Enzyme:** Adenylosuccinate synthetase and lyase
  - o **Energy source:** GTP
- **GMP synthesis:** IMP + NAD^+ + ATP + Glutamine → XMP → GMP
  - o **Enzymes:** IMP dehydrogenase, GMP synthetase
  - o **Energy source:** ATP
- **Regulation:** Reciprocal regulation ensures balanced AMP and GMP levels.

5. Salvage Pathway

- Recycles free purine bases (adenine, guanine, hypoxanthine) to nucleotides using **PRPP**.
- **Enzymes**
  - o Hypoxanthine-guanine phosphoribosyltransferase (HGPRT)
  - o Adenine phosphoribosyltransferase (APRT)
- **Clinical relevance:** Deficiency in HGPRT leads to **Lesch-Nyhan**

syndrome, causing uric acid accumulation and neurological problems.

B. Biosynthesis of Pyrimidine Nucleotides

Pyrimidine nucleotides include **cytosine (C), uracil (U), and thymine (T)**. The key difference from purines is that **the pyrimidine ring is synthesized first**, and then attached to **PRPP** to form nucleotides.

1. Formation of Carbamoyl Phosphate

- **Substrates:** Glutamine + CO_2 + 2 ATP
- **Enzyme:** Carbamoyl phosphate synthetase II (CPS II, cytosolic, rate-limiting)
- **Reaction:** Glutamine + CO_2 + 2 ATP → Carbamoyl phosphate + 2 ADP + Pi
- **Regulation**
    - Inhibited by UTP (feedback inhibition)
    - Activated by PRPP

2. Formation of Carbamoyl Aspartate

- **Substrates:** Carbamoyl phosphate + Aspartate
- **Enzyme:** Aspartate transcarbamoylase (ATCase, committed step)
- **Reaction:** Carbamoyl phosphate + Aspartate → Carbamoyl aspartate

3. Cyclization to Dihydroorotate

- **Enzyme:** Dihydroorotase
- **Reaction:** Carbamoyl aspartate → Dihydroorotate (ring closure forms pyrimidine ring)

4. Oxidation to Orotate

- **Enzyme:** Dihydroorotate dehydrogenase
- **Reaction:** Dihydroorotate → Orotate
- **Significance:** Orotate is the pyrimidine ring precursor.

5. Formation of Orotidine Monophosphate (OMP)

- **Substrates:** Orotate + PRPP → Orotidine monophosphate (OMP)
- **Enzyme:** Orotate phosphoribosyltransferase
- **Significance:** Ribose phosphate attached to orotate, forming the

nucleotide.

6. Formation of UMP, UDP, UTP, and CTP

- **OMP → UMP:** Ornitidylate decarboxylase removes CO_2
- **UMP → UDP → UTP:** Sequential phosphorylation using ATP
- **UTP → CTP:** Glutamine provides amino group
  - **Enzyme:** CTP synthetase
  - **Reaction:** UTP + Glutamine + ATP → CTP + Glutamate + ADP + Pi

7. Formation of dTMP (Deoxythymidine Monophosphate)

- **Substrate:** dUMP (from UDP → dUDP → dUMP)
- **Enzyme:** Thymidylate synthase
- **Cofactor:** N5,N10-methylene tetrahydrofolate
- **Reaction:** dUMP + N5,N10-methylene-THF → dTMP + dihydrofolate
- **Significance:** Provides thymidine for DNA synthesis.

Catabolism of Purine Nucleotides

Purine catabolism is the biochemical process by which purine nucleotides—**adenine, guanine, hypoxanthine, and xanthine**—are degraded to **uric acid**, which is excreted in urine. This pathway maintains nucleotide balance, prevents accumulation of toxic intermediates, and provides nitrogen for excretion. The catabolism involves **removal of phosphate groups, cleavage of ribose, deamination, oxidation, and formation of uric acid**.

A. Degradation of AMP (Adenosine Monophosphate)

1. **Conversion of AMP to Adenosine**
   - **Enzyme:** 5′-Nucleotidase
   - **Reaction:** AMP → Adenosine + Pi
   - **Significance:** Removes phosphate to generate a nucleoside.
2. **Deamination of Adenosine to Inosine**
   - **Enzyme:** Adenosine deaminase (ADA)
   - **Reaction:** Adenosine + H_2O → Inosine + NH_3

- **Significance:** Introduces a keto group at C6, converting adenine to hypoxanthine precursor.

3. **Cleavage of Inosine to Hypoxanthine**
   - **Enzyme:** Purine nucleoside phosphorylase (PNP)
   - **Reaction:** Inosine + Pi → Hypoxanthine + Ribose-1-phosphate
   - **Significance:** Removes the ribose sugar to yield the free purine base hypoxanthine.

B. Degradation of GMP (Guanosine Monophosphate)

1. **Conversion of GMP to Guanosine**
   - **Enzyme:** 5′-Nucleotidase
   - **Reaction:** GMP → Guanosine + Pi
2. **Cleavage of Guanosine to Guanine**
   - **Enzyme:** Purine nucleoside phosphorylase (PNP)
   - **Reaction:** Guanosine + Pi → Guanine + Ribose-1-phosphate
3. **Deamination of Guanine to Xanthine**
   - **Enzyme:** Guanine deaminase
   - **Reaction:** Guanine + H_2O → Xanthine + NH_3

C. Conversion of Hypoxanthine and Xanthine to Uric Acid

1. **Oxidation of Hypoxanthine to Xanthine**
   - **Enzyme:** Xanthine oxidase
   - **Reaction:** Hypoxanthine + H_2O + O_2 → Xanthine + H_2O_2
2. **Oxidation of Xanthine to Uric Acid**
   - **Enzyme:** Xanthine oxidase
   - **Reaction:** Xanthine + H_2O + O_2 → Uric acid + H_2O_2

- **Significance:** Uric acid is the final, relatively insoluble end product in humans and is excreted primarily in urine.

D. Purine Salvage Pathway

The **salvage pathway** recycles purine bases and nucleosides to synthesize nucleotides, conserving energy and preventing excessive uric acid formation.

1. **Hypoxanthine and Guanine Salvage**

o **Enzyme:** Hypoxanthine-guanine phosphoribosyltransferase (HGPRT)

o **Reaction:**

▪ Hypoxanthine + PRPP → IMP + PPi

▪ Guanine + PRPP → GMP + PPi

2. **Adenine Salvage**

o **Enzyme:** Adenine phosphoribosyltransferase (APRT)

o **Reaction:** Adenine + PRPP → AMP + PPi

- **Clinical relevance:** Deficiency of HGPRT leads to **Lesch-Nyhan syndrome**, characterized by hyperuricemia, self-mutilation, and neurological defects.

E. Regulation of Purine Catabolism

1. **Xanthine oxidase activity:** Inhibited by **allopurinol**, a structural analog of hypoxanthine, used to treat gout.

2. **Feedback control:** AMP and GMP levels regulate their own synthesis and degradation.

3. **Salvage pathway efficiency:** Ensures minimal accumulation of free purine bases, preventing excessive uric acid formation.

F. Clinical Significance of Purine Catabolism

1. **Hyperuricemia and Gout:** Excess uric acid precipitates as **monosodium urate crystals**, causing arthritis and kidney stones.

2. **Lesch-Nyhan Syndrome:** X-linked recessive disorder due to **HGPRT deficiency**, leading to uric acid overproduction.

3. **Immunodeficiency: Adenosine deaminase deficiency** results in accumulation of toxic metabolites, causing **Severe Combined Immunodeficiency (SCID)**.

4. **Pharmacological Targets**

o **Allopurinol:** inhibits xanthine oxidase to reduce uric acid levels in gout.

o **Febuxostat:** non-purine xanthine oxidase inhibitor.

Hyperuricemia

Hyperuricemia is defined as an abnormally elevated level of **uric acid** in the blood. In humans, normal uric acid levels are approximately **3.5–7.2 mg/dL in men** and **2.6–6.0 mg/dL in women**. Hyperuricemia occurs when the **production of uric acid exceeds its excretion** or when excretion is impaired, leading to urate accumulation in blood and tissues.

Causes of Hyperuricemia: Hyperuricemia can be classified based on its underlying mechanism:

1. Increased Production of Uric Acid

- **Excessive purine intake:** High consumption of purine-rich foods such as meat, seafood, and organ meats.
- **Increased nucleotide turnover:** Conditions with high cell turnover like **leukemia, psoriasis, or hemolytic anemia** increase purine catabolism.
- **Genetic enzyme defects:**

o **Lesch-Nyhan syndrome:** HGPRT deficiency increases uric acid formation due to impaired salvage of hypoxanthine and guanine.

o **PRPP synthetase overactivity:** Leads to increased purine synthesis and uric acid production.

2. Decreased Excretion of Uric Acid

- **Renal insufficiency:** Chronic kidney disease reduces uric acid excretion.
- **Drugs that impair urate excretion:**

o Diuretics (thiazides, loop diuretics)

o Low-dose aspirin

o Cyclosporine

- **Genetic defects in renal transporters:** Mutations in **URAT1 or GLUT9** transporters reduce uric acid clearance.

Pathophysiology of Hyperuricemia

- **Uric acid accumulation** in blood → formation of **monosodium urate crystals**
- Crystals deposit in:
  - **Joints** → triggers **gouty arthritis**
  - **Kidneys** → causes **urate nephropathy** and **renal calculi**
- **Inflammatory response:** Urate crystals are recognized by macrophages, activating the **NLRP3 inflammasome**, leading to **IL-1β release** and joint inflammation.

Clinical Manifestations

1. Gout

- **Acute gouty arthritis:** Sudden onset of severe pain, redness, swelling, and warmth, commonly in the **first metatarsophalangeal joint (podagra)**.
- **Chronic gout:** Formation of **tophi** (urate crystal deposits) in joints, cartilage, and soft tissues.

2. Renal Complications

- **Urate nephrolithiasis:** Kidney stones composed of uric acid.
- **Chronic urate nephropathy:** Progressive renal damage due to crystal deposition.

3. Asymptomatic Hyperuricemia: Many individuals have elevated uric acid levels without symptoms, but are at risk for developing gout or kidney disease.

Diagnosis of Hyperuricemia

- **Serum uric acid measurement:** Confirms elevated levels.
- **24-hour urinary uric acid excretion:** Differentiates between **overproduction** and **under-excretion**.
- **Imaging:** Ultrasound or X-ray may show urate crystals in joints or tophi.
- **Synovial fluid analysis:** Needle-shaped, negatively birefringent crystals under polarized light microscopy confirm gout.

Management of Hyperuricemia

1. Lifestyle and Dietary Modifications

- Limit intake of **purine-rich foods**: meat, liver, sardines, anchovies, and seafood.
- Increase **water intake** to promote uric acid excretion.
- Limit **alcohol consumption**, especially beer.
- Maintain a **healthy body weight** and avoid rapid weight loss.

2. Pharmacological Treatment

- **Uricostatics (decrease uric acid production)**
  - **Allopurinol:** Inhibits **xanthine oxidase**, reducing uric acid synthesis.
  - **Febuxostat:** Non-purine selective xanthine oxidase inhibitor.
- **Uricosurics (increase uric acid excretion)**
  - **Probenecid, Lesinurad:** Increase renal clearance of urate by inhibiting reabsorption.
- **Acute gout management**
  - **NSAIDs (e.g., indomethacin, naproxen)** for pain and inflammation.
  - **Colchicine:** Reduces crystal-induced inflammation.
  - **Corticosteroids:** Used in severe attacks or when NSAIDs are contraindicated.

Complications of Hyperuricemia

- **Tophi formation:** Permanent joint deformities due to chronic deposition of urate crystals.
- **Uric acid nephrolithiasis:** Leads to kidney stones and urinary obstruction.
- **Chronic kidney disease:** Resulting from persistent urate deposition in renal tissue.
- **Increased cardiovascular risk:** Hyperuricemia is associated with hypertension, metabolic syndrome, and atherosclerosis.

Gout Disease

Gout is a metabolic disorder characterized by the **deposition of monosodium urate (MSU) crystals** in joints, soft tissues, and kidneys, resulting from **persistent hyperuricemia**. It is a type of inflammatory arthritis and is commonly referred to as the **"disease of kings"** due to its association with rich diets. Gout is more common in men than women and typically manifests in middle age.

Etiology of Gout: Gout arises from **increased uric acid levels** due to either **overproduction** or **underexcretion**. The main causes include:

1. Primary Gout (Idiopathic)

- Most cases are due to **genetic predisposition** affecting purine metabolism or renal urate handling.
- **Enzyme defects**
    - **HGPRT deficiency** → Lesch-Nyhan syndrome
    - **PRPP synthetase overactivity** → increased purine synthesis

2. Secondary Gout (Acquired)

- **Increased purine load:** Rapid cell turnover, hemolytic anemia, leukemia, psoriasis
- **Renal insufficiency:** Reduced uric acid excretion
- **Drugs:** Thiazide diuretics, loop diuretics, low-dose aspirin, cyclosporine
- **Dietary factors:** High intake of red meat, seafood, and alcohol (especially beer)

Pathophysiology of Gout

1. **Hyperuricemia:** Persistent high uric acid levels in blood.
2. **Crystal formation:** Supersaturation of uric acid leads to **monosodium urate (MSU) crystal precipitation**.
3. **Inflammatory response**
    - MSU crystals are phagocytosed by **macrophages**, activating the **NLRP3 inflammasome.**
    - **Interleukin-1β (IL-1β)** and other cytokines are released, attracting neutrophils and causing intense inflammation.

4. Tissue deposition: Crystals deposit in joints (especially lower extremities), cartilage, tendons, and kidneys, causing **tophi and renal complications**.

Clinical Features of Gout

1. Acute Gouty Arthritis

- Sudden onset of severe pain, often at **night**.
- Commonly affects **first metatarsophalangeal joint (podagra)**.
- Signs: redness, warmth, swelling, and tenderness.
- Fever and malaise may occur in severe attacks.

2. Intercritical Period

- Symptom-free intervals between acute attacks.
- Hyperuricemia persists silently.

3. Chronic Tophaceous Gout

- Repeated attacks lead to formation of **tophi**, which are firm deposits of MSU crystals in joints, cartilage, and soft tissues.
- Tophi can cause **joint deformity, stiffness, and disability**.

4. Renal Manifestations

- **Uric acid nephrolithiasis:** Kidney stones formed from urate crystals.
- **Chronic urate nephropathy:** Progressive renal dysfunction due to crystal deposition.

Diagnosis of Gout

1. Serum uric acid measurement: Elevated uric acid levels (>7 mg/dL in men, >6 mg/dL in women).

2. Synovial fluid analysis: Needle-shaped, negatively birefringent crystals under polarized light microscopy.

3. Radiological examination: X-rays may show **joint erosion and tophi** in chronic gout.

4. 24-hour urine uric acid: Differentiates **overproduction** from **under-excretion**.

Management of Gout

1. Lifestyle and Dietary Measures

- Restrict **purine-rich foods** (meat, seafood, organ meats).
- Increase **fluid intake** to enhance uric acid excretion.
- Limit **alcohol consumption**, especially beer.
- Maintain a **healthy body weight**.

2. Pharmacological Treatment

- **Acute attack management**

o **NSAIDs:** Indomethacin, naproxen, or diclofenac reduce pain and inflammation.

o **Colchicine:** Inhibits neutrophil migration and crystal-induced inflammation.

o **Corticosteroids:** Used if NSAIDs or colchicine are contraindicated.

- **Chronic urate-lowering therapy**

o **Allopurinol:** Xanthine oxidase inhibitor that reduces uric acid production.

o **Febuxostat:** Non-purine xanthine oxidase inhibitor.

o **Uricosuric agents:** Probenecid, lesinurad increase renal excretion of uric acid.

Complications of Gout

1. **Tophi formation:** Permanent joint deformities due to chronic urate deposits.
2. **Renal stones:** Urate stones causing obstruction or infection.
3. **Chronic kidney disease:** Progressive renal impairment from crystal deposition.
4. **Cardiovascular risk:** Hyperuricemia associated with hypertension, metabolic syndrome, and atherosclerosis.

Organization of Mammalian Genome

The **genome** of an organism refers to the **entire set of genetic material**, including all DNA sequences that encode functional genes and regulatory elements. In mammals, the genome is organized in a highly structured and hierarchical manner to efficiently store, replicate, and express genetic information. Understanding genome organization is essential for grasping genetic regulation, inheritance, and molecular biology.

Components of the Mammalian Genome

1. DNA

o The primary component of the genome, composed of nucleotides with four nitrogenous bases: **adenine (A), guanine (G), cytosine (C), and thymine (T).**

o DNA exists as **double-stranded helical molecules** that encode genetic information.

2. Genes

o Functional units of heredity that code for **proteins or functional RNAs.**

o Mammalian genomes contain approximately **20,000–25,000 protein-coding genes.**

o Genes consist of **exons** (coding sequences) and **introns** (non-coding sequences).

3. Regulatory Sequences

o **Promoters:** DNA regions upstream of genes that initiate transcription.

o **Enhancers and silencers:** Control the level and timing of gene expression.

o **Insulators:** Prevent inappropriate interactions between regulatory elements and genes.

4. Non-coding DNA

o Includes **introns, repetitive sequences, transposable elements, and non-coding RNAs.**

o Plays roles in **chromatin organization, gene regulation, and genome stability.**

Chromosomal Organization: Mammalian DNA is packaged into **chromosomes**, which are highly structured to fit inside the nucleus.

1. Chromosome Structure

- **Chromatin:** DNA is complexed with **histone and non-histone proteins** to form chromatin.
- **Nucleosome:** The fundamental unit of chromatin, consisting of **147 bp of DNA wrapped around an octamer of histone proteins (H2A, H2B, H3, H4)**.
- **Higher-order folding:** Nucleosomes coil into **30 nm fibers**, which further fold into loops and domains to form **chromosomes** during interphase.

2. Chromosome Types in Mammals

- Mammals are **diploid**, containing two sets of chromosomes (2n).
- Chromosomes are classified as:
  - **Autosomes:** Numbered 1–22, containing most of the genetic material.
  - **Sex chromosomes:** X and Y, determining sex and carrying sex-linked genes.
- Each chromosome has distinct regions:
  - **Telomeres:** Protective ends preventing DNA degradation.
  - **Centromeres:** Essential for proper chromosome segregation during mitosis and meiosis.
  - **P and Q arms:** Short (p) and long (q) arms of the chromosome.

Nuclear DNA Organization

1. **Euchromatin**
   - Loosely packed chromatin, transcriptionally active.
   - Contains most **expressed genes**.
2. **Heterochromatin**
   - Densely packed chromatin, transcriptionally inactive.
   - Found in **telomeres, centromeres, and repetitive regions**.
   - Includes **constitutive heterochromatin** (always silent) and **facultative heterochromatin** (conditionally silent).
3. **Topologically Associating Domains (TADs)**
   - Functional domains of chromatin that **regulate interactions between enhancers and promoters**.

Mitochondrial Genome

- Mammals also contain a **small circular DNA molecule** in mitochondria.
- Approximately **16.5 kb in humans**, encoding **13 proteins, 22 tRNAs, and 2 rRNAs**.
- Inherited **maternally**.

Organization of Genes in the Genome

1. **Coding Sequences (Exons)**
   - Contain sequences that are translated into proteins.
2. **Non-coding Sequences (Introns)**
   - Spliced out during mRNA processing.
   - Can regulate gene expression and mRNA stability.
3. **Repetitive DNA Elements**
   - **Tandem repeats:** Satellites, minisatellites, microsatellites.
   - **Interspersed repeats:** LINEs (Long Interspersed Nuclear Elements), SINEs (Short Interspersed Nuclear Elements).
   - Play roles in **chromosome structure, evolution, and genome plasticity**.

Functional Organization

- **Gene density:** Varies across chromosomes; gene-rich regions are transcriptionally active, while gene-poor regions are heterochromatic.
- **Replication origins:** Multiple sites allow rapid DNA replication.
- **Epigenetic modifications:** DNA methylation and histone modifications regulate **gene expression and chromatin structure.**

Structure of DNA

DNA is the genetic material in most organisms and exists mainly as a **double-stranded helix.**

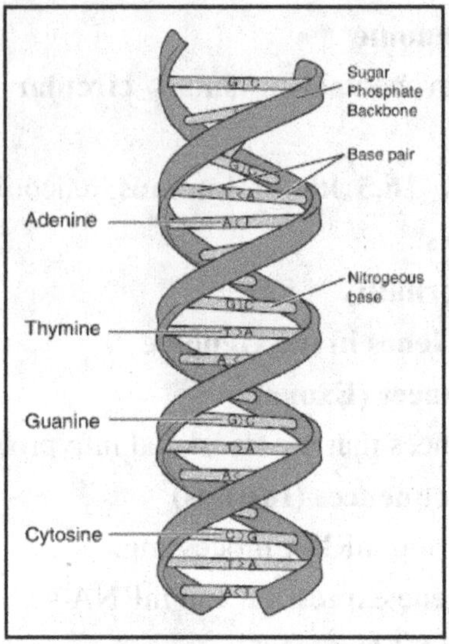

Fig; Structure of DNA

Chemical Composition of DNA

- **Nucleotides:** The basic units of DNA, each consisting of:

1. Deoxyribose: A five-carbon sugar lacking a hydroxyl group at the 2′ position.

2. Nitrogenous base: Purines **(adenine, guanine)** and pyrimidines (**cytosine, thymine**).

3. Phosphate group: Links nucleotides via phosphodiester bonds.

- **Polynucleotide formation:** Nucleotides are joined via **3′–5′ phosphodiester bonds**, forming a sugar-phosphate backbone.

Double Helix Structure (Watson-Crick Model)

- **Strands:** Two antiparallel polynucleotide chains (5′→3′ and 3′→5′).
- **Base pairing**
    - Adenine (A) pairs with Thymine (T) via **2 hydrogen bonds**
    - Guanine (G) pairs with Cytosine (C) via **3 hydrogen bonds**
- **Helical parameters**
    - Right-handed helix **(B-DNA)**

- 10 base pairs per turn
- Helical diameter: ~2 nm
- Major and minor grooves provide binding sites for proteins

- **Stability:** Hydrogen bonding and base stacking interactions stabilize the DNA helix.

Types of DNA

- **A-DNA:** Right-handed helix, shorter and wider, dehydrated form.
- **B-DNA:** Most common form in cells, right-handed helix.
- **Z-DNA:** Left-handed helix, found in some regulatory regions.

Functions of DNA

1. **Storage of genetic information:** Encodes instructions for protein and RNA synthesis.
2. **Transmission of genetic information:** Replicates accurately during cell division.
3. **Template for transcription:** DNA serves as a template to synthesize RNA.
4. **Regulation of gene expression:** DNA sequences control gene activation and silencing.
5. **Evolutionary role:** Mutations in DNA provide genetic diversity.

Structure of RNA

RNA is usually single-stranded and plays key roles in gene expression.

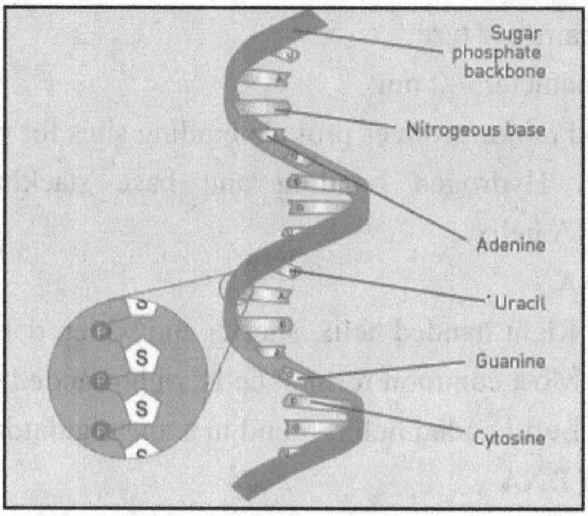

Fig; Structure of RNA

Chemical Composition of RNA

- **Nucleotides:** Each nucleotide contains:

1. **Ribose:** Five-carbon sugar with hydroxyl groups at both 2′ and 3′ positions.
2. **Nitrogenous base:** Purines (**adenine, guanine**) and pyrimidines (**cytosine, uracil**) – **thymine is replaced by uracil (U)**.
3. **Phosphate group:** Forms the backbone via phosphodiester linkages.

- **Polynucleotide formation:** Nucleotides are joined by **3′–5′ phosphodiester bonds**, forming a sugar-phosphate backbone.

Types of RNA and Their Structures

1. **Messenger RNA (mRNA)**
   - o Linear, carries genetic information from DNA to ribosomes for protein synthesis.
   - o Contains **codons** specifying amino acids.
2. **Ribosomal RNA (rRNA)**
   - o Forms the core of ribosome structure and catalyzes peptide bond formation.
   - o Folds into complex secondary and tertiary structures.

3. **Transfer RNA (tRNA)**

o Cloverleaf structure with anticodon region and amino acid attachment site.

o Transfers amino acids to ribosomes during translation.

4. **Other RNAs**

o Small nuclear RNA (snRNA), microRNA (miRNA), small interfering RNA (siRNA) – involved in **RNA splicing, gene regulation, and RNA interference**.

Functions of RNA

1. **Protein synthesis**
   - o **mRNA** carries the genetic code.
   - o **tRNA** brings amino acids.
   - o **rRNA** forms ribosomes and catalyzes peptide bond formation.
2. **Regulation of gene expression**
   - o **miRNA and siRNA** regulate transcription and translation.
3. **Catalytic activity**

o Some RNA molecules **(ribozymes)** catalyze biochemical reactions, e.g., self-splicing introns.

4. **Genetic material in some viruses**

o RNA serves as the **genome of retroviruses and RNA viruses**.

Differences between DNA and RNA

Feature	DNA	RNA
Sugar	Deoxyribose	Ribose
Strands	Double-stranded	Single-stranded
Bases	A, G, C, T	A, G, C, U
Stability	Stable, less reactive	Less stable, more reactive
Function	Genetic storage, transmission	Protein synthesis, regulation, catalysis
Location	Mainly nucleus	Nucleus and cytoplasm

DNA Replication (Semi-Conservative Model)

DNA replication is the biological process by which a cell duplicates its DNA prior to cell division, ensuring that each daughter cell receives an **identical copy of genetic information**. It is a highly regulated, accurate process involving multiple enzymes and proteins.

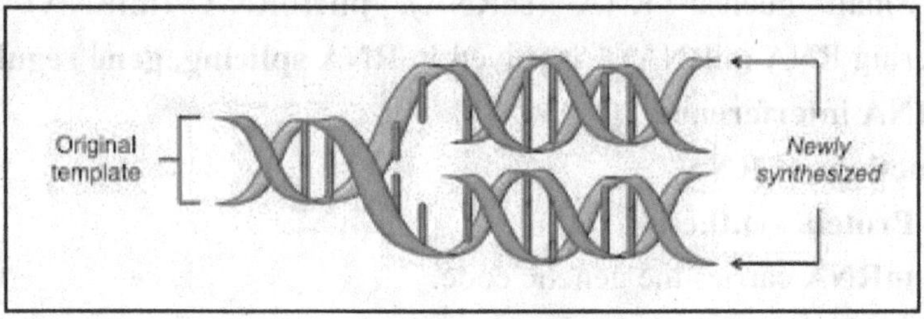

Fig; DNA Replication

Features of DNA Replication

1. **Semi-conservative nature:** Each daughter DNA molecule consists of **one parental strand** and **one newly synthesized strand**.
2. **Directionality:** DNA synthesis occurs in the **5′ → 3′ direction.**
3. **Origin of replication:** Replication begins at specific sequences called **origins of replication** (Ori).
4. **Bidirectional synthesis:** DNA replication is usually bidirectional, forming replication **forks.**
5. **Requirement of primers:** DNA polymerase requires a **short RNA primer** to initiate synthesis.

Semi-Conservative Model of DNA Replication

The **semi-conservative model** was experimentally demonstrated by **Meselson and Stahl (1958)** using **isotopes of nitrogen (^{15}N and ^{14}N)** in E. coli:

1. **Experimental setup**

- E. coli grown in heavy nitrogen (^{15}N) incorporated it into DNA.
- Bacteria were then shifted to light nitrogen (^{14}N) medium and

allowed to replicate.

2. **Results**

o After one generation, DNA molecules had intermediate density (hybrid of ^{15}N and ^{14}N).

o After two generations, DNA molecules consisted of **half hybrid (^{15}N-^{14}N)** and **half light (^{14}N-^{14}N)**.

3. **Conclusion**

o Each daughter DNA consists of **one parental strand** and **one newly synthesized strand**, confirming the **semi-conservative nature** of DNA replication.

Mechanism of DNA Replication

Replication involves **initiation, elongation, and termination** steps, occurring in the **S-phase of the cell cycle** in eukaryotes.

1. Initiation

- **Origin recognition:** Replication begins at **Ori sites**.
- **Helicase:** Unwinds the double helix, creating a **replication fork**.
- **Single-strand binding proteins (SSB):** Stabilize unwound DNA strands.
- **Topoisomerase (Gyrase):** Relieves supercoiling ahead of the fork.
- **Primase:** Synthesizes a short **RNA primer** complementary to the template strand.

2. Elongation

- **DNA polymerase III (prokaryotes) / DNA polymerases δ and ε (eukaryotes):** Adds nucleotides **5′ → 3′**, complementary to the template strand.
- **Leading strand synthesis:** Continuous synthesis toward the replication fork.
- **Lagging strand synthesis:** Discontinuous synthesis away from the fork forming **Okazaki fragments**.
- **Primer removal and replacement:**

- **DNA polymerase I (prokaryotes) / RNase H and DNA polymerase δ (eukaryotes)** remove RNA primers and replace them with DNA.

- **DNA ligase:** Seals gaps between Okazaki fragments, forming a continuous strand.

3. Termination

- Replication ends when **replication forks meet** or at **termination sequences** in prokaryotes.
- In eukaryotes, linear chromosome ends are maintained by **telomerase**, which adds repetitive sequences to prevent loss of genetic material.

Transcription (RNA Synthesis)

Transcription is the process by which **genetic information encoded in DNA is copied into RNA**. It is the first step in **gene expression** and occurs in both **prokaryotic and eukaryotic cells**. The RNA synthesized can be **messenger RNA (mRNA), ribosomal RNA (rRNA), transfer RNA (tRNA), or other non-coding RNAs.**

Features of Transcription

1. **Template-directed synthesis:** Only one DNA strand, called the **template strand**, is used to synthesize RNA.
2. **Directionality:** RNA synthesis occurs in the **5′ → 3′ direction**.
3. **Complementarity:** RNA bases are complementary to DNA template bases:
   - A (DNA) → U (RNA), T (DNA) → A (RNA), G ↔ C.
4. **No primer required:** Unlike DNA replication, RNA polymerase **initiates synthesis de novo.**

Types of RNA Synthesized

1. **Messenger RNA (mRNA):** Carries genetic code from DNA to ribosomes for protein synthesis.
2. **Ribosomal RNA (rRNA):** Forms the structural and catalytic core of ribosomes.

3. Transfer RNA (tRNA): Brings amino acids to ribosomes during translation.

4. Other RNAs: Small nuclear RNA (snRNA), microRNA (miRNA), small interfering RNA (siRNA) – involved in **RNA processing, gene regulation, and RNA interference.**

Mechanism of Transcription

Transcription occurs in **three main steps: initiation, elongation, and termination.**

1. Initiation

- **Promoter recognition:** RNA polymerase binds to a **promoter region** upstream of the gene.
  - **Prokaryotes:** σ-factor helps RNA polymerase recognize the -10 (TATAAT) and -35 regions.
  - **Eukaryotes:** Transcription factors bind to **TATA box** and other regulatory sequences to recruit RNA polymerase II (for mRNA).
- **DNA unwinding:** RNA polymerase unwinds the DNA helix to expose the **template strand.**
- **Start of RNA synthesis:** RNA polymerase synthesizes the first few nucleotides of RNA complementary to the DNA template.

Elongation

- RNA polymerase moves along the DNA template strand **3′ → 5′**, adding ribonucleotides in the **5′ → 3′ direction.**
- DNA **rewinds behind the polymerase**, forming a transient **transcription bubble.**
- The **nascent RNA strand** grows complementary to the DNA template strand.

Termination

- **Prokaryotic termination**
  - **Rho-independent:** Hairpin loop in RNA followed by a series of U residues causes polymerase release.
  - **Rho-dependent:** Rho protein moves along RNA and disrupts the RNA-DNA complex.

- **Eukaryotic termination**
  - RNA polymerase II transcribes past the **polyadenylation signal (AAUAAA).**
  - RNA is cleaved and processed with a **5′ cap and 3′ poly-A tail.**

RNA Processing (Eukaryotes)

1. **5′ Capping:** Addition of **7-methylguanosine** protects mRNA from degradation and aids in ribosome binding.
2. **3′ Polyadenylation:** Addition of a **poly-A tail** stabilizes mRNA and facilitates export from the nucleus.
3. **Splicing:** Removal of **introns** and joining of **exons** by spliceosomes to form mature mRNA.

Regulation of Transcription

- **Promoters and enhancers:** Control gene-specific expression.
- **Transcription factors:** Proteins that activate or repress transcription.
- **Epigenetic modifications:** DNA methylation and histone modifications influence transcriptional activity.

Functions of Transcription

1. **Synthesis of RNA:** Provides templates for **protein synthesis**.
2. **Gene expression regulation:** Determines which genes are expressed in different tissues or conditions.
3. **Production of functional RNAs:** rRNA, tRNA, snRNA, and regulatory RNAs are synthesized.
4. **Basis for cell differentiation and adaptation:** Transcription controls protein production necessary for specific cellular functions.

Genetic Code

The **genetic code** is the set of rules by which the sequence of **nucleotides in DNA or RNA** is translated into the **sequence of amino acids in a protein**. It provides the molecular basis for converting genetic information into functional proteins, ensuring the correct synthesis of polypeptides in all living organisms.

Features of the Genetic Code

1. **Triplet nature**

o The genetic code consists of **three nucleotide bases (codon)** that specify **one amino acid**.

o Example: AUG codes for Methionine.

2. **Comma-less**

o Codons are read **continuously without punctuation**; there are no gaps between codons.

3. **Non-overlapping**

o Each nucleotide is part of **only one codon**, ensuring precise translation.

4. **Degeneracy (redundancy)**

o Most amino acids are encoded by **more than one codon**.

o Example: Leucine is coded by six codons (UUA, UUG, CUU, CUC, CUA, CUG).

5. **Universal nature**

o The genetic code is nearly **universal**, conserved across prokaryotes and eukaryotes, with few minor exceptions in mitochondria.

6. **Start and stop signals**

o **Start codon (AUG):** Signals initiation of translation and codes for Methionine.

o **Stop codons (UAA, UAG, UGA):** Signal termination of protein synthesis.

7. **Specificity:**

o Each codon specifies **only one amino acid** or a termination signal.

Codons and Their Types

1. **Sense codons:** Codons that specify amino acids (61 out of 64).
2. **Nonsense codons (stop codons):** Do not code for amino acids but terminate translation (UAA, UAG, UGA).
3. **Start codon:** AUG, which codes for Methionine and signals the **initiation of translation**.

Wobble Hypothesis

- Proposed by **Francis Crick**, the wobble hypothesis explains **degeneracy in the genetic code.**
- The **3rd base of the codon** can pair less strictly with the **1st base of the anticodon** in tRNA.
- Example: G in the anticodon can pair with C or U in the codon.
- Significance: Reduces the number of tRNAs required and allows flexibility in base pairing.

Characteristics of the Genetic Code

Feature	Description
Triplet	3 nucleotides = 1 codon = 1 amino acid
Universal	Same in almost all organisms
Degenerate	Most amino acids are specified by multiple codons
Non-overlapping	Each nucleotide belongs to only one codon
Start/Stop	AUG = start, UAA/UAG/UGA = stop
Comma-less	Read continuously without breaks
Specific	Each codon codes for only one amino acid

Significance of Genetic Code

1. **Accurate protein synthesis:** Ensures correct sequence of amino acids in polypeptides.
2. **Genetic fidelity:** Prevents errors during translation, maintaining cellular function.
3. **Universality:** Allows genetic engineering and expression of genes across species.
4. **Redundancy protection:** Degeneracy minimizes effects of point mutations (silent mutations).

5. **Basis for molecular biology techniques:** Used in **gene cloning, recombinant DNA technology, and synthetic biology**.

Translation (Protein Synthesis) and Its Inhibitors

Translation is the process by which the **genetic information carried by mRNA** is decoded to synthesize a **specific polypeptide or protein**. It occurs in the **cytoplasm** at the ribosomes and involves multiple RNA molecules and protein factors.

Features of Translation

1. **Template-directed synthesis:** mRNA serves as a template specifying the amino acid sequence.
2. **Directionality:** Polypeptide synthesis occurs in the **N-terminal to C-terminal direction**.
3. **Codon recognition:** Each codon on mRNA corresponds to a specific amino acid, read by **tRNA anticodons**.
4. **Energy-dependent:** Requires **GTP and ATP** for tRNA charging and peptide bond formation.

Components of Translation

1. **mRNA**
   - Carries the genetic code from DNA.
   - Contains **start codon (AUG), codons for amino acids, and stop codon**.
2. **tRNA**
   - Transfers amino acids to the ribosome.
   - Has an **anticodon** complementary to mRNA codon and an **amino acid attachment site**.
3. **Ribosomes**
   - **Prokaryotes:** 70S ribosome (50S + 30S subunits)
   - **Eukaryotes:** 80S ribosome (60S + 40S subunits)
   - Contains **A (aminoacyl), P (peptidyl), and E (exit) sites** for tRNA binding.

4. Aminoacyl-tRNA synthetases

- o Enzymes that charge tRNAs with the correct amino acid using ATP.

5. Translation factors

- o **Initiation factors (IFs), elongation factors (EFs), release factors (RFs)** aid in initiation, elongation, and termination.

Stages of Translation

1. Initiation

- Ribosomal subunits assemble on **mRNA** at the **start codon (AUG)**.
- **Prokaryotes:** Initiator tRNA carries **formyl-methionine (fMet)**.
- **Eukaryotes:** Initiator tRNA carries **methionine (Met)**.
- Initiation factors position the ribosome correctly to start translation.

2. Elongation

- **Aminoacyl-tRNA binding:** tRNA binds to the **A site** of the ribosome.
- **Peptide bond formation:** Catalyzed by **peptidyl transferase** in the ribosome; bond forms between N-terminal of the new amino acid and C-terminal of the growing chain.
- **Translocation:** Ribosome moves one codon along mRNA, shifting tRNAs from **A → P → E site**.

3. Termination

- Occurs when ribosome reaches a **stop codon (UAA, UAG, UGA)**.
- **Release factors (RFs)** promote hydrolysis of the polypeptide from tRNA.
- Ribosomal subunits, mRNA, and tRNA dissociate, completing translation.

Inhibitors of Translation

Several drugs inhibit translation by targeting **different stages or components** of protein synthesis.

Drug	Target/Mechanism	Effect
Streptomycin	30S ribosomal subunit (prokaryotes)	Misreading of mRNA, inhibits initiation
Tetracycline	30S ribosomal subunit	Blocks aminoacyl-tRNA binding to A site
Chloramphenicol	50S ribosomal subunit	Inhibits peptidyl transferase, preventing peptide bond formation
Erythromycin / Macrolides	50S ribosomal subunit	Prevents translocation of ribosome along mRNA
Puromycin	Resembles aminoacyl-tRNA	Causes premature chain termination
Cycloheximide	Eukaryotic 80S ribosome	Inhibits peptidyl transferase, blocks elongation
Actinomycin D	DNA/RNA hybrid	Prevents mRNA synthesis (indirectly inhibits translation)

Functions and Significance of Translation

1. **Protein synthesis:** Converts genetic code into functional proteins essential for cellular structure and function.
2. **Gene expression:** Final step in the central dogma (DNA → RNA → Protein).
3. **Cellular regulation:** Enables cells to respond to environmental changes by synthesizing necessary proteins.
4. **Biotechnological applications:** Understanding translation is crucial for **recombinant protein production, antibiotics, and molecular biology research**.

Chapter-8

Enzymes

Enzymes are biological catalysts that play a crucial role in accelerating chemical reactions within living organisms without being consumed in the process. They are predominantly proteins, although some RNA molecules, known as ribozymes, also exhibit catalytic activity. Enzymes are highly specific in their action, meaning that each enzyme typically catalyzes only one type of chemical reaction or acts on a particular substrate. This specificity is a result of the unique three-dimensional structure of the enzyme, which allows precise binding with its substrate at the active site.

Enzymes function by lowering the activation energy required for a chemical reaction, thereby increasing the reaction rate significantly. This is essential for sustaining life because many biochemical reactions are too slow under physiological conditions to meet the needs of cells and tissues without enzymatic catalysis. Enzymes are involved in a wide range of physiological processes including metabolism, DNA replication, signal transduction, and energy production.

The study of enzymes, known as enzymology, includes understanding their structure, mechanism of action, kinetics, regulation, and their applications in medicine, industry, and research. Enzymes are also sensitive to environmental conditions such as pH, temperature, and the presence of inhibitors or activators, which can influence their activity.

Properties of Enzymes

Enzymes exhibit several distinctive properties that differentiate them from ordinary chemical catalysts and define their functionality in biological systems. These properties are crucial for understanding enzyme behavior, mechanism of action, and their applications in medicine and industry. The main properties of enzymes include:

1. Catalytic Efficiency

Enzymes are highly efficient catalysts, capable of increasing the rate of biochemical reactions by several million-fold compared to uncatalyzed reactions. This high catalytic efficiency ensures that metabolic processes occur rapidly enough to sustain life under physiological conditions.

2. Specificity

Enzymes display two types of specificity:

- **Substrate Specificity:** Each enzyme typically acts on a particular substrate or a group of closely related substrates. For example, sucrase specifically catalyzes the hydrolysis of sucrose.
- **Reaction Specificity:** Enzymes are also specific for the type of reaction they catalyze. For instance, oxidoreductases catalyze oxidation-reduction reactions, while transferases transfer functional groups.

3. Active Site Requirement

The activity of an enzyme depends on the presence of an active site, a specially shaped region that binds the substrate. The three-dimensional structure of the active site allows precise interaction with the substrate through weak forces such as hydrogen bonds, ionic interactions, and van der Waals forces.

4. Reversibility

Enzymes can catalyze both the forward and reverse reactions, depending on the concentrations of substrates and products, thus maintaining metabolic equilibrium. The direction of the reaction is governed by the principle of thermodynamic equilibrium.

5. Sensitivity to Environmental Conditions

Enzyme activity is affected by factors such as pH, temperature, and ionic strength:

- **pH:** Each enzyme has an optimal pH at which it exhibits maximum activity. Deviations can alter the ionization state of amino acid residues at the active site and reduce activity.
- **Temperature:** Enzymes have an optimal temperature; higher

temperatures may denature the enzyme, while lower temperatures decrease the reaction rate.

- **Ionic Strength:** High salt concentrations can affect enzyme stability and substrate binding.

6. Regulation

Enzymes are subject to regulation by activators and inhibitors, allowing cells to control metabolic pathways according to physiological needs. This property is essential for maintaining homeostasis.

7. Reusability

Enzymes are not consumed in the reactions they catalyze. After the reaction, they are regenerated in their original form, making them reusable for multiple reaction cycles.

8. High Molecular Weight

Most enzymes are proteins with high molecular weight, which contributes to their complex three-dimensional structure and functional specificity.

9. Stereospecificity

Enzymes can distinguish between different stereoisomers of a substrate, catalyzing the reaction of one specific isomer while ignoring others. This property is particularly important in biochemical pathways involving chiral molecules.

10. Activation Energy Reduction

Enzymes accelerate reactions by lowering the activation energy, which is the minimum energy required to initiate a chemical reaction. This allows reactions to occur under mild physiological conditions.

Nomenclature of Enzymes

The nomenclature of enzymes is a systematic way of naming enzymes based on the type of reaction they catalyze and their substrate specificity. Proper naming helps in classifying enzymes, understanding their function, and facilitating communication among scientists and researchers. The nomenclature is governed by the **International Union**

of Biochemistry and Molecular Biology (IUBMB).

1. Systematic Nomenclature

In systematic nomenclature, the name of an enzyme is derived from the substrate it acts on followed by the type of reaction it catalyzes. This provides clear information about both the substrate and the reaction. For example:

- **Lactase:** Catalyzes the hydrolysis of lactose into glucose and galactose.
- **Alcohol dehydrogenase:** Catalyzes the oxidation of alcohol to aldehyde or ketone.

The systematic name often ends with the suffix **"-ase,"** which is characteristic of enzymes.

2. Common or Trivial Names

Many enzymes were discovered before the standard nomenclature system was established and are known by common or trivial names. These names are widely used and often reflect the substrate, source, or historical context rather than the reaction type. Examples include:

- **Pepsin:** A protease found in the stomach.
- **Trypsin:** A pancreatic enzyme that hydrolyzes proteins.
- **Lipase:** An enzyme that hydrolyzes lipids.

3. IUBMB Classification System (EC Number)

The International Union of Biochemistry and Molecular Biology (IUBMB) has introduced a numerical classification system for enzymes called the **Enzyme Commission (EC) number**. Each enzyme is assigned a unique EC number consisting of four parts, which classify the enzyme based on the reaction it catalyzes:

EC X.X.X.X

- **First digit:** Denotes the main class of enzyme according to the type of reaction catalyzed. There are six major classes:

1. **Oxidoreductases:** Catalyze oxidation-reduction reactions.
2. **Transferases:** Transfer functional groups from one molecule to another.

3. **Hydrolases:** Catalyze hydrolysis reactions.

4. **Lyases:** Catalyze the addition or removal of groups to form double bonds.

5. **Isomerases:** Catalyze structural rearrangements within a molecule.

6. **Ligases:** Catalyze the joining of two molecules using energy from ATP.

- **Second digit:** Specifies the subclass, detailing the type of bond or group involved.
- **Third digit:** Indicates the sub-subclass, giving more specificity about the substrate or reaction.
- **Fourth digit:** A serial number identifying the particular enzyme within the sub-subclass.

For example:

- **EC 1.1.1.1** — Alcohol dehydrogenase (oxidoreductase acting on the CH–OH group with NAD+ or NADP+ as acceptor).

Enzyme Kinetics

Enzyme kinetics is the study of the rate at which enzyme-catalyzed reactions occur and how these rates change with varying substrate concentrations, enzyme concentrations, and environmental conditions. Understanding enzyme kinetics is essential to characterize enzyme behavior, determine enzyme efficiency, and design inhibitors or drugs that target specific enzymes. Two fundamental concepts in enzyme kinetics are the **Michaelis-Menten kinetics** and the **Lineweaver-Burk plot.**

1. Michaelis-Menten Kinetics

The Michaelis-Menten model describes the relationship between the rate of an enzyme-catalyzed reaction and substrate concentration. It assumes that the enzyme (E) binds reversibly to the substrate (S) to form an enzyme-substrate complex (ES), which then converts into the product (P) and regenerates the free enzyme. The reaction can be represented as:

$E + S \rightleftharpoons ES \rightarrow E + P$

Key assumptions of the Michaelis-Menten model:

- The formation of the enzyme-substrate complex is rapid and reaches a steady-state.
- The breakdown of the enzyme-substrate complex to product is the rate-limiting step.
- Substrate concentration is much higher than enzyme concentration.

Michaelis-Menten Equation: The rate of the reaction (v) is given by:

V = Vmax [S] / Km + [S]

Where:

- **v** = initial velocity of the reaction
- **Vmax** = maximum reaction velocity when the enzyme is saturated with substrate
- **[S]** = substrate concentration
- **Km** = Michaelis constant, the substrate concentration at which the reaction rate is half of Vmax

Significance of Michaelis-Menten parameters

- **Vmax** indicates the catalytic efficiency of the enzyme when fully saturated with substrate.
- **Km** reflects the affinity of the enzyme for its substrate: a lower Km indicates higher affinity, while a higher Km indicates lower affinity.

Michaelis-Menten Plot: The Michaelis-Menten plot is a hyperbolic curve obtained by plotting reaction velocity (v) against substrate concentration ([S]). At low substrate concentration, the reaction rate increases almost linearly with [S], but at higher [S], the rate approaches V_{max} asymptotically, indicating enzyme saturation. This plot helps visualize how enzymes respond to varying substrate concentrations.

2. Lineweaver-Burk Plot (Double Reciprocal Plot)

The Lineweaver-Burk plot is a linear transformation of the Michaelis-Menten equation, which makes it easier to determine kinetic parameters (Vmax and Km) graphically. By taking the reciprocal of both sides of the

Michaelis-Menten equation:

$$\frac{1}{V_0} = \frac{K_m}{V_{max}}\left(\frac{1}{[S]}\right) + \frac{1}{V_{max}}$$

This equation is in the form **y = mx + c**, where:

- **y = 1/v** (reciprocal of reaction velocity)
- **x = 1/[S]** (reciprocal of substrate concentration)
- **Slope (m) = Km / Vmax**
- **Y-intercept = 1 / Vmax**
- **X-intercept = -1 / Km**

Significance of Lineweaver-Burk Plot

- Provides a precise method to calculate Vmax and Km.
- Facilitates analysis of enzyme inhibition, including competitive, non-competitive, and uncompetitive inhibition, as different types of inhibition produce characteristic changes in the plot.
- Converts the hyperbolic Michaelis-Menten relationship into a straight line, simplifying data interpretation.

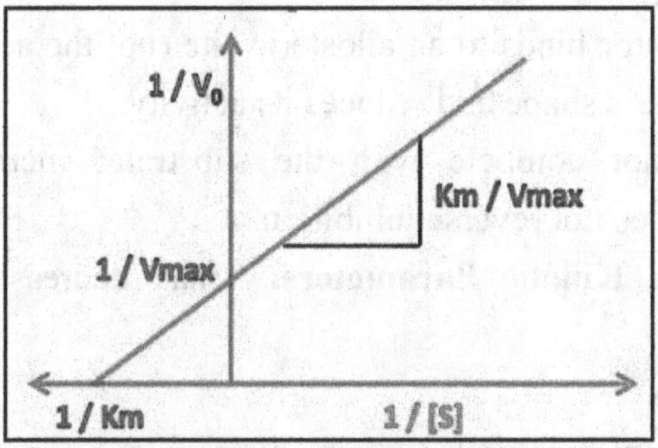

Enzyme Inhibitors

Enzyme inhibitors are molecules that decrease or completely block the activity of an enzyme. They play a crucial role in regulating metabolic pathways, controlling enzyme activity in vivo, and serving as drugs or therapeutic agents. Inhibitors can act reversibly or irreversibly, depending on how they interact with the enzyme.

Classification of Enzyme Inhibitors: Enzyme inhibitors are broadly classified into **reversible** and **irreversible** inhibitors.

A. Reversible Inhibitors

These inhibitors bind non-covalently to the enzyme and can dissociate, allowing the enzyme to regain its activity. Reversible inhibition is further categorized based on how the inhibitor interacts with the enzyme or enzyme-substrate complex:

i. Competitive Inhibition

- The inhibitor competes with the substrate for binding at the enzyme's active site.
- It resembles the substrate's structure and can be overcome by increasing substrate concentration.
- **Effect on Kinetic Parameters:** Vmax remains unchanged; Km increases.
- **Examples**
  - **Methotrexate** inhibits dihydrofolate reductase.
  - **Malonate** inhibits succinate dehydrogenase.

ii. Non-Competitive Inhibition

- The inhibitor binds to an allosteric site (not the active site), which alters the enzyme's shape and reduces its activity.
- It does not compete with the substrate; increasing substrate concentration does not reverse inhibition.
- **Effect on Kinetic Parameters:** Vmax decreases; Km remains unchanged.
- **Examples**
  - **Phenylalanine** inhibits tyrosine hydroxylase.
  - **Heavy metals** like lead (Pb^{2+}) inhibit enzymes such as ALAD in heme synthesis.

iii. Uncompetitive Inhibition

- The inhibitor binds only to the enzyme-substrate complex, preventing the formation of the product.

- **Effect on Kinetic Parameters:** Both Vmax and Km decrease.
- **Examples**
  - **Lithium ions** inhibiting inositol monophosphatase.
  - Some inhibitors of alkaline phosphatase.

B. Irreversible Inhibitors

Irreversible inhibitors bind covalently to the enzyme, permanently inactivating it. Recovery of enzyme activity requires new enzyme synthesis.

Examples

- **Aspirin:** Acetylates cyclooxygenase (COX) enzyme, permanently inhibiting prostaglandin synthesis.
- **Penicillin:** Inhibits transpeptidase in bacterial cell wall synthesis.
- **Diisopropylfluorophosphate (DFP):** Irreversibly inhibits serine proteases and acetylcholinesterase.

Physiological and Pharmacological Significance of Enzyme Inhibitors

- **Regulation of Metabolism:** Natural inhibitors control metabolic pathways by feedback inhibition. For example, ATP inhibits phosphofructokinase in glycolysis.
- **Drug Design:** Many drugs function as enzyme inhibitors, such as ACE inhibitors (captopril) for hypertension and protease inhibitors for HIV therapy.
- **Toxin Mechanism:** Certain toxins act as enzyme inhibitors, e.g., cyanide inhibits cytochrome oxidase in the electron transport chain.

Regulation of Enzymes

Enzyme regulation refers to the processes by which cells control the activity, specificity, and amount of enzymes to ensure that metabolic pathways function efficiently and respond to the physiological needs of the organism. Proper regulation of enzymes is essential for maintaining homeostasis, preventing wasteful reactions, and coordinating complex metabolic processes. Enzyme regulation occurs at multiple levels, including genetic control, allosteric regulation, covalent modification, and environmental factors.

Enzyme Induction: Enzyme induction refers to the **increase in the synthesis of an enzyme** in response to the presence of a specific substrate or molecule. Induction ensures that enzymes are produced only when their substrate is available, preventing unnecessary energy expenditure.

Mechanism of Enzyme Induction

- When the substrate (inducer) is present, it binds to a repressor or regulatory protein, causing a conformational change.
- This prevents the repressor from binding to the DNA, allowing transcription of the enzyme's gene.
- As a result, the enzyme is synthesized in increased amounts.

Examples of Enzyme Induction

- **β-Galactosidase:** In *E. coli*, lactose induces the production of β-galactosidase by inactivating the lac repressor.
- **Cytochrome P450 enzymes:** In liver cells, certain drugs (e.g., phenobarbital) induce the production of cytochrome P450 enzymes, enhancing drug metabolism.
- **Alcohol dehydrogenase:** Ethanol can induce its own metabolism by increasing enzyme synthesis in some organisms.

Physiological Significance of Enzyme Induction

- Allows cells to respond to the availability of substrates.
- Conserves energy by synthesizing enzymes only when required.
- Plays a role in drug metabolism and detoxification.

Enzyme Repression: Enzyme repression refers to the **decrease or inhibition of enzyme synthesis** in response to the accumulation of an end product or a regulatory molecule. This prevents overproduction of enzymes and conserves cellular resources.

Mechanism of Enzyme Repression

- The end product or co-repressor binds to a regulatory protein (repressor).

- The repressor then binds to the operator region of the DNA, blocking transcription of the enzyme gene.
- Consequently, enzyme synthesis is reduced or halted.

Examples of Enzyme Repression

- **Tryptophan synthetase:** In *E. coli*, high levels of tryptophan repress the synthesis of enzymes involved in tryptophan biosynthesis.
- **Arginine biosynthesis enzymes:** Arginine acts as a co-repressor to inhibit the enzymes in its biosynthetic pathway.

Physiological Significance of Enzyme Repression

- Prevents accumulation of unnecessary enzymes and metabolites.
- Maintains metabolic homeostasis.
- Conserves energy and cellular resources by halting unneeded enzyme production.

Regulation of Allosteric Enzymes: Allosteric enzymes are a special class of enzymes whose activity is regulated by molecules that bind to sites other than the active site, called **allosteric sites**. These enzymes are usually involved in key regulatory steps of metabolic pathways and are capable of fine-tuning metabolic flux in response to cellular needs. Allosteric regulation is a rapid and reversible way to control enzyme activity.

Characteristics of Allosteric Enzymes

- **Multiple Subunits:** Most allosteric enzymes are oligomeric proteins composed of multiple subunits, each containing an active site.
- **Allosteric Site:** Apart from the active site, these enzymes possess one or more allosteric sites where regulatory molecules (effectors) bind.
- **Sigmoidal Kinetics:** Unlike typical Michaelis-Menten enzymes that exhibit a hyperbolic relationship between reaction velocity and substrate concentration, allosteric enzymes show **sigmoidal (S-shaped) kinetics**, reflecting cooperative interactions between subunits.
- **Cooperativity:** Binding of substrate or effector to one subunit affects the affinity or activity of other subunits. Positive cooperativity enhances substrate binding at other sites, while negative cooperativity

reduces it.

Types of Allosteric Regulation

A. Allosteric Activation

- Activators bind to the allosteric site and stabilize the enzyme in its **active (R) conformation**, increasing its catalytic activity.
- Activators may increase substrate affinity or enhance the rate of catalysis.
- **Example:** AMP activates phosphofructokinase-1 (PFK-1) in glycolysis, signaling low energy status and promoting glucose metabolism.

B. Allosteric Inhibition

- Inhibitors bind to the allosteric site and stabilize the enzyme in its **inactive (T) conformation**, decreasing activity.
- This mechanism often prevents unnecessary accumulation of pathway intermediates.
- **Example:** ATP and citrate inhibit PFK-1, signaling sufficient energy and slowing glycolysis.

Mechanism of Allosteric Regulation

Two major models explain allosteric regulation:

i. Concerted Model (MWC Model)

- All subunits of the enzyme exist in either the **tense (T, low affinity)** or **relaxed (R, high affinity)** state.
- Binding of substrate or activator shifts the equilibrium toward the R state, increasing activity.
- Inhibitors shift the equilibrium toward the T state.

ii. Sequential Model (KNF Model)

- Subunits change conformation sequentially upon ligand binding.
- Binding of substrate or effector to one subunit induces conformational changes in neighboring subunits, affecting their activity.

Physiological Importance of Allosteric Enzyme Regulation

- Provides precise control of key metabolic pathways such as glycolysis, gluconeogenesis, and the citric acid cycle.

- Enables rapid response to changes in substrate or energy levels.
- Prevents accumulation of intermediates and ensures metabolic balance.
- Serves as the basis for **feedback inhibition**, a common regulatory mechanism where the end product of a pathway inhibits an allosteric enzyme at an early step.

Examples of Allosteric Enzymes and Regulation

- **Phosphofructokinase-1 (PFK-1):** Activated by AMP, inhibited by ATP and citrate.
- **Aspartate transcarbamoylase (ATCase):** Inhibited by CTP, activated by ATP.
- **Glycogen phosphorylase:** Activated by AMP, inhibited by ATP and glucose-6-phosphate.

Coenzymes

Coenzymes are **organic, non-protein molecules** that are essential for the catalytic activity of certain enzymes. Unlike cofactors, which may be inorganic ions, coenzymes participate in enzyme-catalyzed reactions by acting as carriers of specific chemical groups or electrons. Coenzymes themselves are not consumed in the reaction but may undergo reversible chemical changes during the catalytic process.

Definition: A coenzyme is a **small organic molecule that binds to an enzyme and assists in catalysis**, often by transferring functional groups (e.g., acyl, methyl, or phosphate groups) or electrons between molecules. Many coenzymes are derived from vitamins, which are essential nutrients that organisms cannot synthesize in sufficient amounts.

Characteristics of Coenzymes

- Organic molecules, often derived from vitamins.
- Required in small amounts.
- Bind temporarily (cosubstrate) or permanently (prosthetic group) to the enzyme.

- Act as carriers of electrons, atoms, or functional groups in biochemical reactions.
- Reusable, as they are regenerated after the reaction.

Types of Coenzymes

A. Cosubstrates

- Bind **loosely** to the enzyme and **participate transiently** in the reaction.
- After the reaction, they are released and regenerated by another enzyme or reaction.
- **Example**
  - **NAD^+ (Nicotinamide adenine dinucleotide):** Carries electrons in oxidation-reduction reactions.
  - **FAD (Flavin adenine dinucleotide):** Transfers electrons in redox reactions.
  - **Coenzyme A (CoA):** Carries acyl groups in metabolic reactions.

B. Prosthetic Groups

- Bind **tightly or covalently** to the enzyme and remain attached during the catalytic cycle.
- Essential for enzyme activity, forming part of the holoenzyme.
- **Example**
  - **FAD** in succinate dehydrogenase.
  - **Biotin** in carboxylase enzymes, carrying CO_2.

Significance of Coenzymes

- Enable enzymes to perform complex chemical transformations that amino acid side chains alone cannot.
- Serve as carriers for electrons, protons, or functional groups.
- Connect metabolic pathways by transferring intermediates.
- Many coenzymes are targets for drug design or nutritional interventions, as deficiencies can impair enzyme function and lead to metabolic disorders.

Structure of Coenzymes

Coenzymes are small organic molecules with **distinct structural**

features that allow them to participate effectively in enzyme-catalyzed reactions. Their structure determines their **binding ability, functional group transfer**, and **electron-carrying capacity**. Most coenzymes are derived from vitamins, and their structures typically include nucleotide components, heterocyclic rings, or reactive functional groups essential for catalysis.

General Structural Features of Coenzymes

- **Organic Molecules:** Composed primarily of carbon, hydrogen, nitrogen, oxygen, and sometimes phosphorus or sulfur.
- **Functional Groups:** Contain reactive groups such as hydroxyl (-OH), amine ($-NH_2$), sulfhydryl (-SH), phosphate ($-PO_4$), or carbonyl (C=O) that participate in chemical reactions.
- **Nucleotide Components:** Many coenzymes contain an adenine nucleotide (adenosine or ADP derivative) that helps them bind to enzymes.
- **Heterocyclic Rings:** Important for electron transfer, as seen in nicotinamide (NAD^+/$NADP^+$) and flavin (FAD/FMN).
- **Flexible Linkers:** Some coenzymes have flexible chains (like pantothenic acid in CoA) that allow them to shuttle functional groups between enzyme active sites.

Structural Examples of Common Coenzymes

A. NAD^+ (Nicotinamide Adenine Dinucleotide)

- Composed of two nucleotides joined by their phosphate groups: one contains **adenine**, the other **nicotinamide**.
- The **nicotinamide ring** is the reactive site, accepting or donating electrons in redox reactions.
- Structure allows **electron transfer** in dehydrogenase-catalyzed reactions.

B. FAD (Flavin Adenine Dinucleotide)

- Contains a **riboflavin (vitamin B2) moiety** attached to an adenine nucleotide.
- The **isoalloxazine ring** is the redox-active portion, capable of

accepting or donating two electrons and two protons.

- The adenine nucleotide helps in **enzyme binding** and proper orientation.

C. Coenzyme A (CoA)

- Composed of **pantothenic acid** linked to **β-mercaptoethylamine** and **adenosine 3′-phosphate**.
- The **terminal sulfhydryl (-SH) group** is the reactive site that forms thioester bonds with acyl groups.
- The structure provides **flexibility** to carry acyl groups in metabolic reactions.

D. Thiamine Pyrophosphate (TPP)

- Derived from **thiamine (Vitamin B1)** with a **pyrophosphate group**.
- Contains a **thiazolium ring**, which acts as the reactive site for decarboxylation of α-keto acids.
- The pyrophosphate allows **binding to enzyme** through interactions with metal ions or amino acid residues.

E. Biotin

- Contains a **ureido ring fused with a tetrahydrothiophene ring**, linked to **valeric acid**.
- The **biotin carboxyl group** forms a covalent bond with CO_2 for carboxylation reactions.
- The long side chain allows **flexible movement** between active sites of multi-enzyme complexes.

F. Pyridoxal Phosphate (PLP)

- Derived from **pyridoxine (Vitamin B6)**.
- Contains an **aldehyde group** that forms a Schiff base with amino groups of amino acids, facilitating transamination and decarboxylation reactions.
- The **aromatic pyridine ring** stabilizes intermediates during catalysis.

Structural Significance

- The **reactive site** (ring, phosphate, sulfhydryl, or aldehyde) participates directly in chemical transformations.
- The **nucleotide or flexible linker** portion ensures proper orientation, binding, and transport of functional groups.
- The specific **three-dimensional structure** allows coenzymes to interact precisely with enzymes and substrates, enhancing catalytic efficiency.

Biochemical Functions of Coenzymes

Coenzymes play a pivotal role in enzymatic reactions by acting as **transient carriers of electrons, atoms, or functional groups**, facilitating chemical transformations that enzymes alone cannot perform. They are essential for numerous metabolic processes, including energy production, biosynthesis, and detoxification. The biochemical functions of coenzymes can be broadly categorized based on the type of chemical reaction they participate in.

1. Electron Transfer (Oxidation-Reduction Reactions)

Some coenzymes act as **electron carriers**, facilitating oxidation-reduction reactions in metabolism. They accept electrons and protons from substrates and donate them to other molecules, enabling the flow of energy in cellular pathways.

- **NAD^+ / $NADP^+$ (Nicotinamide adenine dinucleotide/phosphate):** Accepts two electrons and one proton to form NADH or NADPH. NAD^+ is primarily used in catabolic reactions (e.g., glycolysis, TCA cycle), while NADPH is used in anabolic reactions (e.g., fatty acid synthesis).
- **FAD / FMN (Flavin adenine dinucleotide / flavin mononucleotide):** Accepts two electrons and two protons to form $FADH_2$ or $FMNH_2$, participating in redox reactions such as those in the electron transport chain.

2. Transfer of Functional Groups

Many coenzymes act as **carriers of specific functional groups**, transferring them between molecules in metabolic reactions.

- **Coenzyme A (CoA):** Transfers acyl groups (e.g., acetyl, fatty acyl) in reactions like the formation of acetyl-CoA in carbohydrate and lipid metabolism.
- **Thiamine pyrophosphate (TPP):** Transfers activated aldehyde groups, crucial for decarboxylation of α-keto acids in carbohydrate metabolism.
- **Tetrahydrofolate (THF):** Transfers one-carbon units (e.g., methyl, methylene, formyl) in amino acid and nucleotide metabolism.
- **Biotin:** Transfers activated CO_2 in carboxylation reactions, such as conversion of acetyl-CoA to malonyl-CoA during fatty acid synthesis.
- **Pyridoxal phosphate (PLP):** Transfers amino groups in transamination reactions and facilitates decarboxylation and racemization of amino acids.

3. Activation of Substrates

Some coenzymes help **activate substrates**, making them more reactive for enzymatic transformation.

- **ATP (Adenosine triphosphate):** Provides energy for phosphorylation reactions, activating substrates in biosynthetic pathways.
- **Coenzyme A (CoA):** Forms thioester bonds with acyl groups, making them high-energy intermediates suitable for subsequent metabolic reactions.

4. One-Carbon Metabolism

Certain coenzymes carry single-carbon units for biosynthetic processes:

- **Tetrahydrofolate (THF):** Transfers one-carbon units in purine, thymidylate, and amino acid biosynthesis.
- **S-Adenosylmethionine (SAM):** Donates methyl groups in methylation reactions, including DNA, RNA, protein, and lipid methylation.

5. Participation in Electron Transport and Energy Production

Some coenzymes are critical components of **mitochondrial electron transport**, linking substrate oxidation to ATP synthesis.

- **NADH and $FADH_2$:** Donate electrons to the electron transport chain, driving oxidative phosphorylation.
- **Coenzyme Q (Ubiquinone):** Transfers electrons between complexes I/II and III in the mitochondrial membrane.

6. Structural Role in Enzyme Complexes

Certain coenzymes act as **prosthetic groups**, tightly bound to enzymes, stabilizing structure and participating directly in catalysis:

- **FAD in succinate dehydrogenase** and **biotin in carboxylases** serve as essential prosthetic groups.

7. Detoxification Reactions

Coenzymes assist in detoxification by aiding the metabolism and elimination of xenobiotics and drugs:

- **NADPH:** Provides reducing power for cytochrome P450 enzymes in drug metabolism.
- **Glutathione (GSH):** Acts with glutathione-dependent enzymes to neutralize reactive oxygen species.

Therapeutic Applications of Enzymes

Enzymes are employed as **biological drugs** or **therapeutic agents** to treat diseases, replace deficient enzymes, or assist in metabolic and pathological processes.

A. Enzyme Replacement Therapy (ERT)

Enzyme replacement therapy is used to **compensate for inherited or acquired enzyme deficiencies** in metabolic disorders. By supplementing the missing or defective enzyme, normal metabolic function can be restored or partially corrected.

- **Examples**
    - **Pompe disease:** Caused by deficiency of acid α-glucosidase (lysosomal enzyme). Therapeutic administration of **alglucosidase alfa**

helps degrade glycogen accumulated in lysosomes, improving muscle function.

- **Gaucher disease:** Caused by deficiency of β-glucocerebrosidase, leading to lipid accumulation in macrophages. **Imiglucerase** replaces the enzyme, reducing organomegaly and bone complications.
- **Lysosomal storage disorders:** Many lysosomal enzymes are administered as recombinant proteins to manage metabolic accumulation.

B. Thrombolytic Therapy (Fibrinolytic Enzymes)

Certain enzymes dissolve **blood clots** (thrombi) and are crucial in treating myocardial infarction, stroke, and deep vein thrombosis. They act by converting plasminogen to plasmin, which degrades fibrin in clots.

- **Examples**
  - **Streptokinase:** Derived from *Streptococcus*, activates plasminogen systemically.
  - **Urokinase:** A human enzyme that directly activates plasminogen, useful in pulmonary embolism and peripheral arterial thrombosis.
  - **Tissue plasminogen activator (tPA):** Recombinant enzyme used intravenously in acute myocardial infarction and ischemic stroke.

C. Digestive Enzyme Therapy

Enzymes are used to **aid digestion** in patients with pancreatic insufficiency or gastrointestinal disorders. These enzymes help hydrolyze macronutrients and improve nutrient absorption.

- **Examples**
  - **Pancreatin:** A mixture of amylase, lipase, and protease; used in cystic fibrosis or chronic pancreatitis.
  - **Lactase:** Administered orally to hydrolyze lactose in patients with lactose intolerance.
  - **Bile salt-stimulating enzymes**: Support fat absorption in biliary disorders.

D. Enzymes for Debridement and Anti-Inflammatory Therapy

Some proteolytic enzymes are applied to wounds, burns, or inflammatory conditions to remove necrotic tissue and reduce inflammation.

- **Examples**
  - **Collagenase:** Breaks down necrotic collagen in ulcers and burns.
  - **Trypsin and Chymotrypsin:** Used in topical or oral formulations to reduce edema and inflammation.

E. Enzymes in Oncology and Cancer Therapy

- **Asparaginase:** Utilized in **acute lymphoblastic leukemia (ALL)**; it degrades asparagine in the blood, depriving leukemic cells, which cannot synthesize it, of this essential amino acid.
- **L-asparaginase therapy** demonstrates how enzymes can be targeted to metabolic vulnerabilities of cancer cells.

F. Enzymes in Drug Production and Biotechnology

- Enzymes facilitate **stereospecific synthesis** and modification of drugs, improving efficacy and reducing side effects.
- Examples include lipases for ester synthesis and proteases for peptide drugs.

Diagnostic Applications of Enzymes

Enzymes serve as **biochemical markers** for disease because their levels in blood, urine, or other fluids often change in response to tissue damage, disease states, or metabolic disorders.

A. Serum Enzymes as Disease Markers

- Tissue-specific enzymes leak into the bloodstream when cells are damaged. Measuring these enzymes aids in diagnosis and monitoring of disease.
- **Examples**
  - **Liver disease**
    - **Alanine aminotransferase (ALT)**: Specific for hepatocellular injury.
    - **Aspartate aminotransferase (AST)**: Elevated in liver and cardiac injury.
    - **Alkaline phosphatase (ALP):** Elevated in cholestasis or bone

disorders.

- **Pancreatic disorders**
  - **Amylase and Lipase:** Elevated in acute pancreatitis.
- **Cardiac disorders**
  - **Creatine kinase (CK) and CK-MB isoenzyme:** CK-MB is highly specific for myocardial infarction.
  - **Troponins:** Although not enzymes, often measured alongside CK-MB.

B. Isoenzymes (Isozymes) in Tissue-Specific Diagnosis

Isoenzymes are **different molecular forms of the same enzyme** that differ in amino acid sequence, kinetics, and tissue distribution. Measuring specific isoenzymes allows **precise localization of tissue damage.**

Examples of Clinically Important Isoenzymes

1. **Creatine Kinase (CK) Isoenzymes**
   - **CK-MM:** Predominant in skeletal muscle; elevated in muscular dystrophy or trauma.
   - **CK-MB:** Predominant in cardiac muscle; elevated in myocardial infarction.
   - **CK-BB:** Found in brain; elevated in CNS injury or tumors.
2. **Lactate Dehydrogenase (LDH) Isoenzymes**
   - **LDH-1:** Heart-specific; elevated after myocardial infarction.
   - **LDH-2:** Major isoenzyme in red blood cells.
   - **LDH-5:** Liver and skeletal muscle; elevated in liver disease.
3. **Alkaline Phosphatase (ALP) Isoenzymes**
   - **Liver ALP:** Elevated in cholestatic liver disease.
   - **Bone ALP:** Elevated in Paget's disease, rickets, or bone metastasis.
   - **Placental ALP:** Increased in pregnancy.

C. Enzyme-Based Diagnostic Assays

- Enzymes are used in **biosensors and laboratory tests** for detecting metabolites or toxins:

- **Glucose oxidase:** Used in glucometers to monitor blood glucose in diabetes.
- **Cholinesterase assays:** Detect exposure to organophosphates or nerve agents.
- **Amylase and lipase assays:** Confirm acute pancreatitis.
- **Lactate dehydrogenase assay:** Measures tissue hypoxia or hemolysis.

www.ingramcontent.com/pod-product-compliance
Lightning Source LLC
Chambersburg PA
CBHW011349230926
51848CB00003B/520
* 9 7 8 8 1 6 9 2 4 4 4 5 9 *